Super–Easy
Type 2 Diabetes
Cookbook for Beginners

Low-Sugar & Tasty Diabetes Recipes and Meal Plans

will Help You Live in A Better Lifestyle

Yolanda Ferry

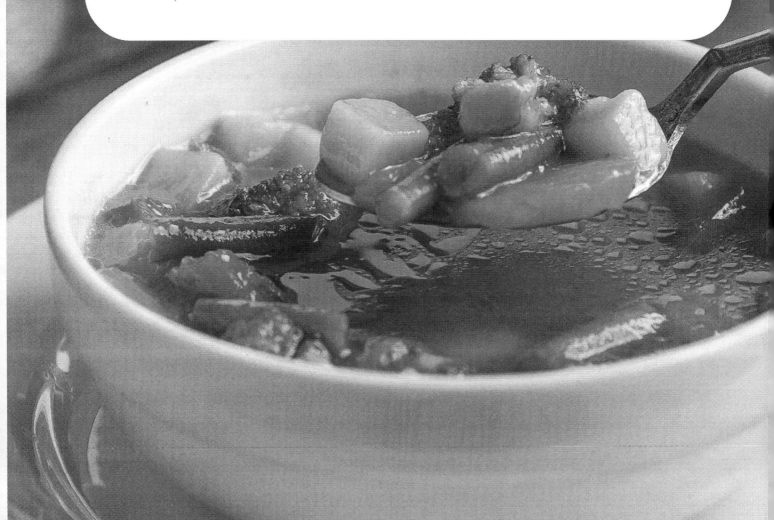

Contents

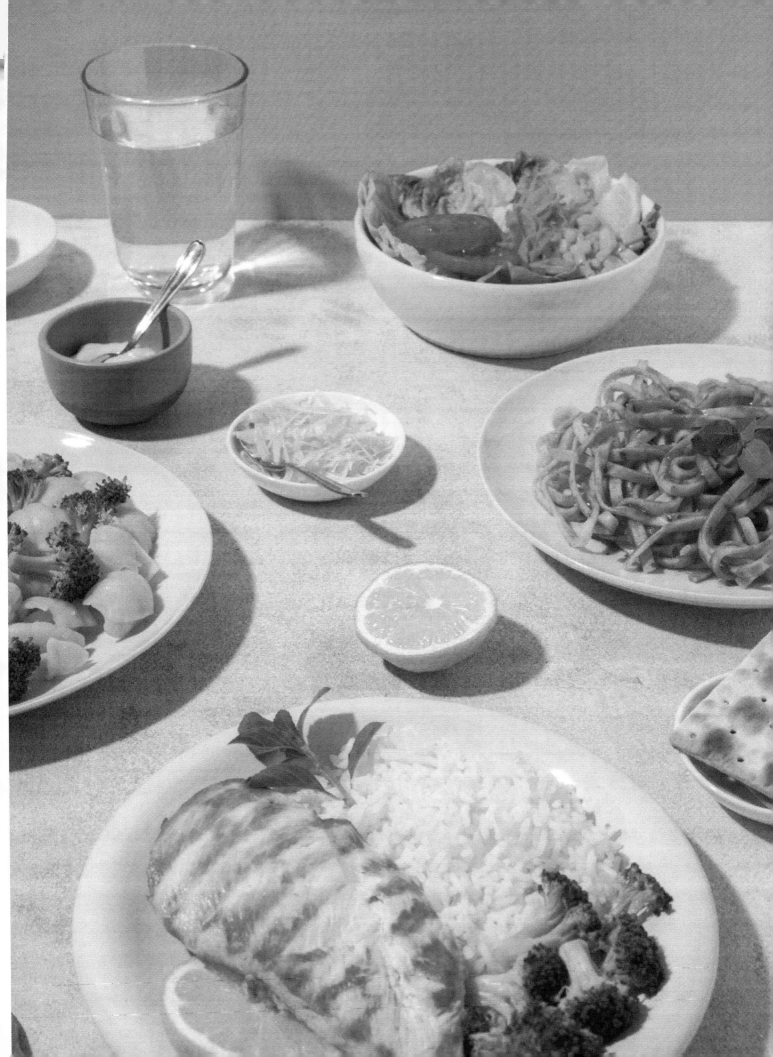

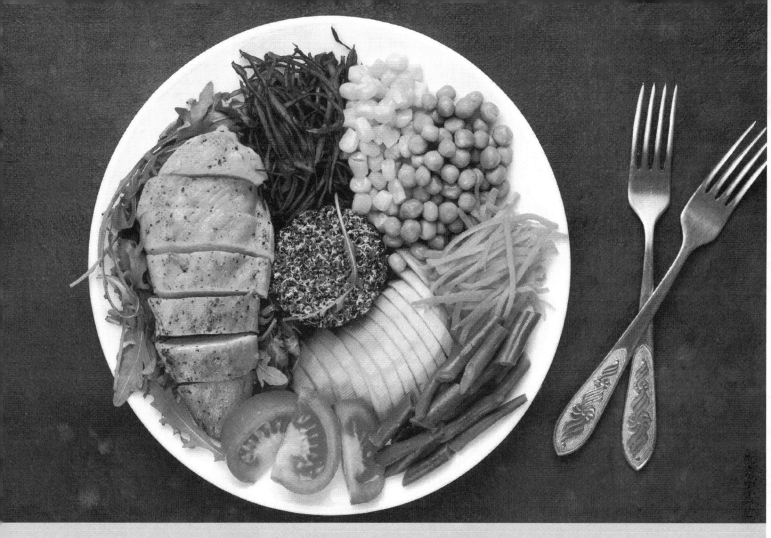

Introduction

The popular saying "Health is wealth" highlights the significance of good health in our lives. However, what happens when you are silently struggling with a chronic illness that can have severe consequences? One such disease is Diabetes, a chronic condition that can go unnoticed for long periods. Diabetes is a condition in which the pancreas either does not produce enough insulin or produces no insulin at all, leading to an increase in blood sugar levels in the body.

There are two types of diabetes: Type 1 and Type 2. Type 1 diabetes is incurable, while Type 2 diabetes can be put in remission with a healthy lifestyle.

Type 2 diabetes mellitus is a chronic metabolic disorder that affects the body's ability to process and utilize sugar (glucose) effectively. This leads to the accumulation of excess sugar in the bloodstream, which can cause damage to blood vessels, nerves, and the immune system over time. Unfortunately, there is currently no cure for type 2 diabetes mellitus, but it can be managed effectively through lifestyle changes such as weight loss, healthy eating, and regular exercise. In some cases, diabetes medication or insulin therapy may also be necessary to help regulate blood sugar levels.

What Is Type 2 diabetes?

Type 2 diabetes mellitus is a chronic metabolic disorder that affects how your body processes glucose, the primary source of energy for your cells. Glucose is obtained from the food you eat and is transported through your bloodstream to your cells with the help of insulin, a hormone produced by the pancreas. In type 2 diabetes, your body either doesn't produce enough insulin or becomes resistant to its effects, leading to a buildup of glucose in your bloodstream. This excess glucose can cause a range of health problems over time, such as nerve damage, kidney failure, vision loss, and cardiovascular disease. It's important to manage type 2 diabetes carefully with medication, lifestyle changes, and regular monitoring to prevent complications and maintain good health.

Some of the symptoms of diabetes include;

- Increased thirst and urination
- Feeling tired
- Increased hunger
- Blurred vision
- Sores that do not heal
- Numbness or tingling in the feet or hands
- Unexplained weight loss

Type 2 diabetes is a chronic condition that affects the way your body processes blood sugar (glucose). The symptoms of this condition usually develop gradually over a period of several years and can be so mild that you might not even notice them. In fact, it's possible that you may not experience any symptoms at all, which is why many people don't even realize they have the condition.

However, if left untreated, type 2 diabetes can lead to serious complications such as heart disease, blindness, kidney failure, and nerve damage. This is why it's important to be aware of the symptoms of type 2 diabetes, which can include frequent urination, increased thirst, increased hunger, fatigue, blurred vision, slow healing of wounds, and numbness or tingling in the hands or feet.

If you experience any of these symptoms, it's important to speak with your healthcare provider right away to get a proper diagnosis and treatment plan. Early diagnosis and treatment of type 2 diabetes can help prevent or delay the onset of complications and improve your overall quality of life.

Differences Between Type-1 and Type-2 Diabetes

It is common for people to have questions about the difference between type 1 and type 2 diabetes, as well as the possibility of developing both conditions. While both types of diabetes share some similarities, there are also several differences that set them apart. To provide some clarity, let's explore the reasons behind each type, who is affected by them, and how they are managed.

Type 1 diabetes is an autoimmune disease that occurs when the immune system mistakenly attacks and kills the insulin-producing cells in the pancreas. This results in little to no insulin production, which is a hormone that regulates blood sugar levels. Type 1 diabetes affects approximately 8% of all diabetics, and it commonly develops in children and young adults.

On the other hand, type 2 diabetes is a metabolic disorder that occurs when the body becomes resistant to insulin or does not produce enough insulin to maintain normal blood sugar levels. Type 2 diabetes is much more prevalent than type 1, accounting for up to 90% of all diabetes cases. It typically develops in adults, although it can occur at any age.

It is important to note that there are other types of diabetes as well, such as gestational diabetes that occurs during pregnancy and maturity-onset diabetes of the young (MODY) that is caused by a genetic mutation.

Managing diabetes involves careful monitoring of blood sugar levels, following a healthy diet, engaging in regular physical activity, and taking medication or insulin as prescribed by a healthcare provider. It is crucial to manage blood sugar levels effectively, as high blood sugar can lead to health problems such as nerve damage, kidney damage, and cardiovascular disease.

If you happen to have both type 1 and type 2 diabetes, it is important to work closely with your healthcare team to develop a personalized management plan that meets your individual needs. Remember, regardless of the type of diabetes you have, managing it effectively is crucial for maintaining good health.

The below table shows some basic knowledge about the type-1 and type-2 Diabetes;

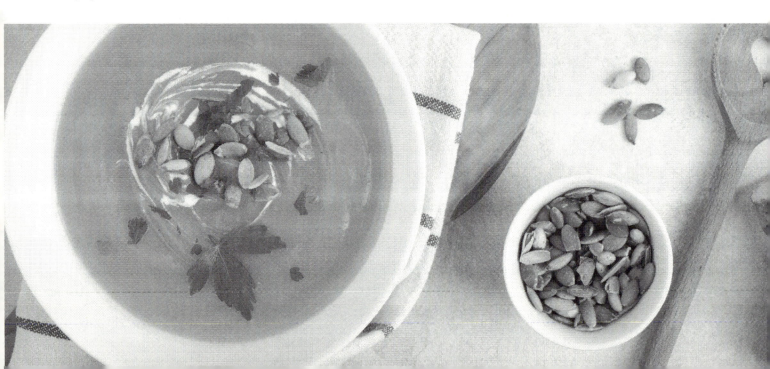

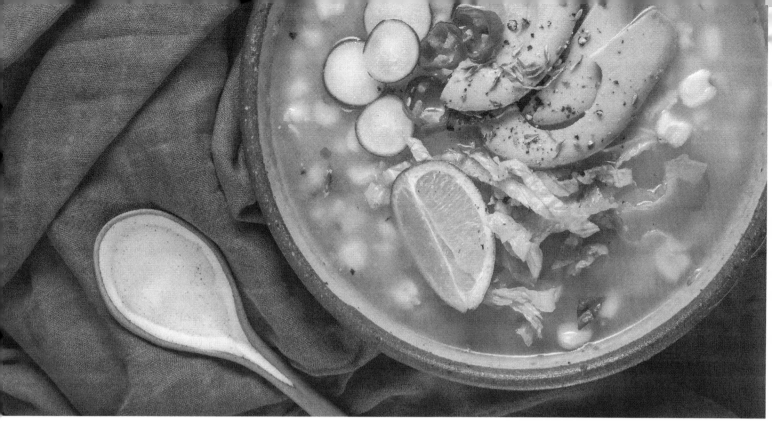

	Type 1 diabetes	Type 2 diabetes
What is happening	Your pancreas is not producing enough insulin to help dissolve glucose in your cells.	The pancreas is producing insulin, but not enough for proper cell function.
Risk Factor	we are currently unaware of any plausible cause for the type-1 incident.	Being obese and belonging to certain ethnic groups increases the risk of developing type-2 diabetes.
Symptoms	The quick appearance of symptoms	Symptoms appearance is mild and slow
How to Manage	Taking insulin is necessary to regulate blood sugar levels	Maintaining a healthy lifestyle through regular exercise such as walking, eating a balanced and nutritious diet, and taking mild medication when necessary is essential for overall wellbeing
Prevention and cure	Not curable	Not curable but can be put into remission with a healthy lifestyle

Type 1 diabetes is an autoimmune disease where the body attacks and destroys the insulin-producing cells. This results in an inability to produce insulin, which is needed to absorb sugar from the blood into the cells for energy. As a result, blood sugar levels become too high.

On the other hand, type 2 diabetes occurs when the body either doesn't produce enough insulin or doesn't use it properly, resulting in insulin resistance. This, in turn, leads to high blood sugar levels, just like in type 1 diabetes.

Formation of Type-2 Diabetes

The risk of developing type 2 diabetes is determined by some factors that can be modified and others that cannot.

◆ Obesity

It is currently unknown why some individuals produce insulin, but it is well-established that obesity and a lack of physical activity can lead to insulin resistance. Improving insulin resistance is crucial in treating and managing type 2 diabetes. Losing weight is one way to improve insulin resistance and manage type 2 diabetes. The location of excess body fat also plays a role in determining the risk of developing type 2 diabetes. Individuals with an "apple" body shape, who carry most of their weight in their stomach area, are at a higher risk of insulin resistance and type 2 diabetes. Conversely, individuals with a "pear" body shape, who carry most of their weight on their hips and thighs, are less likely to develop insulin resistance and type 2 diabetes.

◆ Gestation Period

Gestational diabetes is a type 2 diabetes that can occur during pregnancy. Researchers believe that hormonal changes during pregnancy, genetics, and lifestyle can cause this condition. The hormones produced by the placenta can activate insulin resistance in women after pregnancy, but most women can produce enough insulin to overcome this resistance. However, some women may not be able to produce enough insulin, leading to gestational diabetes mellitus. This condition is also associated with obesity, which can be avoided by maintaining a healthy weight during pregnancy. Excessive weight gain during pregnancy can also lead to gestational diabetes. Hormonal changes, weight gain, and family history can all contribute to gestational diabetes, but it is often temporary and resolves after delivery.

◆ Hypertension

High blood pressure, also known as hypertension, can be a contributing factor to the development of type 2 diabetes. Diabetes mellitus and kidney infections are among the many types of diabetes that can be caused or worsened by hypertension. Moreover, individuals with diabetes are at a higher risk of developing high blood pressure, as well as other heart and circulatory problems. Diabetes can damage the arteries and make them more susceptible to hardening, a condition known as arteriosclerosis. This can lead to high blood pressure that, if left untreated, can result in complications such as blood vessel damage, kidney failure, and heart attack.

The combination of high blood pressure and type 2 diabetes is particularly dangerous and can significantly increase the risk of heart disease or stroke. Diabetic retinopathy can also lead to blindness. Although some people can improve their type 2 diabetes and high blood pressure through lifestyle changes, most require medication. Depending on their overall health, some people may need more than one medication to manage their blood pressure.

◆ Other Causes

Genetic mutations, NIH external link, other, damage to the pancreas, and certain medicines may also cause diabetes.

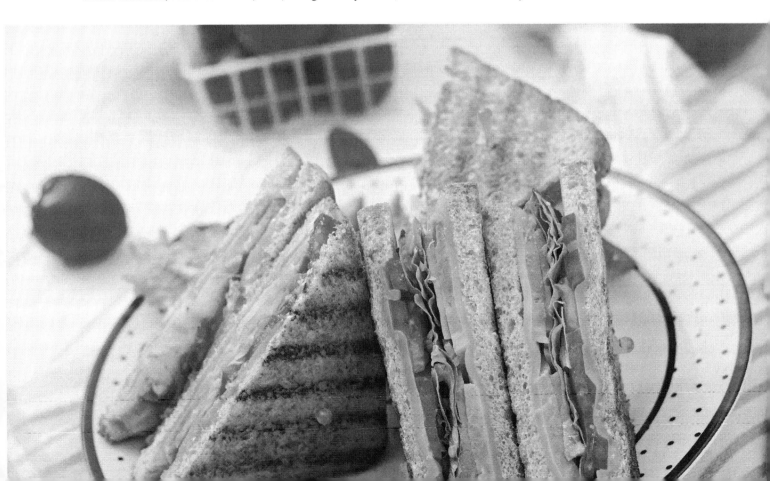

Genes and Family History

It has been found that women with a family history of gestational diabetes are more susceptible to developing the condition. This suggests that genetics play a role in the development of gestational diabetes, which is more common among certain ethnic groups like African Americans, American Indians, Asians, and Hispanics. Diabetes, in general, can be caused by a genetic mutation or change in a gene that affects insulin levels. These mutations are usually inherited, but can also happen spontaneously. When insulin levels drop, it can lead to diabetes. There are different types of diabetes, such as type 1 diabetes which is more common in children, mature-onset diabetes mellitus (MODY), and neonatal diabetes which develops at 6 months of age. Hemochromatosis and cystic fibrosis are two other conditions that can cause diabetes by preventing the pancreas from producing enough insulin due to excess iron or thick mucus buildup. If left untreated, these conditions can lead to further complications.

◆ Hormonal Diseases

Diabetes results from a hormonal imbalance in the body. The pancreas produces insulin, which is absorbed into the blood by fat, muscle, and liver cells for energy and other metabolic processes. In type 2 diabetes, the body resists insulin, so the pancreas produces more insulin to lower blood sugar, but the excess insulin is not stored. This leads to uncontrolled diabetes.

For instance, hormonal changes during menopause can affect blood sugar levels and cause faster changes in postmenopausal women with diabetes. The weight gain during pregnancy may require adjustments in blood sugar levels, while low hormones can disrupt sleep, making it challenging to control blood sugar. Women with diabetes are also more prone to experience sexual problems due to vaginal cell damage caused by the disease.

Men also face similar issues when their body produces low testosterone, such as decreased sex drive and muscle loss. However, many people are unaware that low testosterone can also cause insulin resistance.

Certain hormonal problems cause the body to produce too many hormones, leading to insulin resistance and diabetes. Cushing's syndrome, caused by an excessive amount of cortisol, also known as the "stress hormone", and acromegaly, caused by excessive hormone production, are some examples. Hyperthyroidism, caused by an overactive thyroid gland, can also lead to insulin resistance.

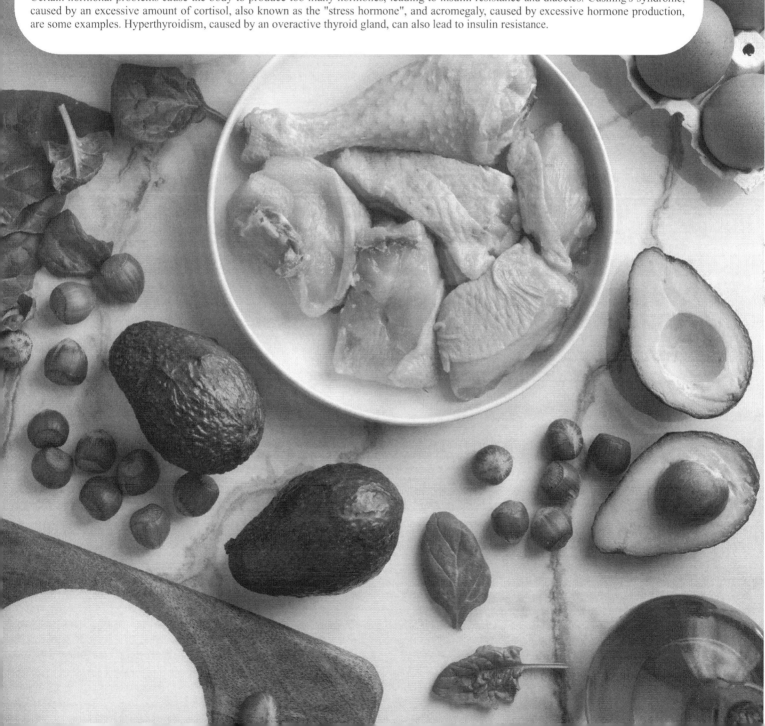

◆ Damage to or Removal of the Pancreas

Pancreatitis, leukemia, and injury can damage beta cells, reducing insulin production and causing diabetes. Eliminating pancreatic cancer can also lead to diabetes due to the loss of beta cells.

How to Prevent and Control Diabetes

If you are at risk of developing diabetes, there are steps you can take to prevent or delay its onset. The most important thing you can do is maintain a healthy lifestyle, which can have additional benefits for your overall health. By making certain changes, you can also reduce your risk of developing other illnesses and improve your overall sense of well-being. Here are some of the changes you can make:

◆ Develop Good Habits

Type-2 diabetes can be put into remission by developing good habits such as maintaining a healthy lifestyle, adopting healthy eating habits, and following proper medication. It is essential to quit smoking and drinking, as these habits can lead to active metabolic activities that worsen diabetes. By managing these activities and adopting a healthy lifestyle, you can reduce the symptoms of diabetes and live a healthy life even with this chronic disease.
Some of the following activities help you to manage type-2 diabetes. Following are:
Cut of refined Carbs and sugar from the diet
It is recommended to avoid certain types of food to lower the risk of developing hypoglycemia. Foods that are high in good carbohydrates and sugar can increase blood sugar and insulin levels, which can lead to this condition. When you consume sugary and carbohydrate-rich foods, your body breaks them down quickly, causing an increase in blood sugar levels. Replacing such foods with healthier alternatives low in carbohydrates can help control diabetes. Individuals who consume large amounts of carbohydrates are at a higher risk of developing type 2 diabetes compared to those who consume less.

◆ Drink a lot of water

Water is considered the most beneficial drink for your health. It helps reduce the risk of diabetes, which can lead to high levels of blood sugar. Studies have shown that drinking water helps the body produce optimal insulin and regulate blood sugar. Moreover, water helps reduce cravings for sugary and salty drinks, which can help maintain healthy blood sugar levels.

◆ Quit Smoking

Smoking is known to increase the risk of diabetes, particularly in those who smoke heavily. Moreover, smoking has been shown to cause or exacerbate serious health conditions, such as heart disease, emphysema, lung cancer, breast cancer, prostate cancer, and indigestion. If you are a smoker, you may be at risk of developing type 2 diabetes. However, quitting smoking can significantly reduce these risks over time.

◆ Take Coffee and Tea

It is important to drink plenty of water, but adding coffee or tea to your diet can also be beneficial in preventing diabetes. Research has shown that daily intake of coffee can reduce the risk of type 2 diabetes, as coffee and tea contain antioxidants known as polyphenols that help prevent diabetes. Green tea, in particular, contains a special antioxidant called epigallocatechin gallate (EGCG) that has been found to reduce the release of blood sugar from the liver and increase insulin secretion.

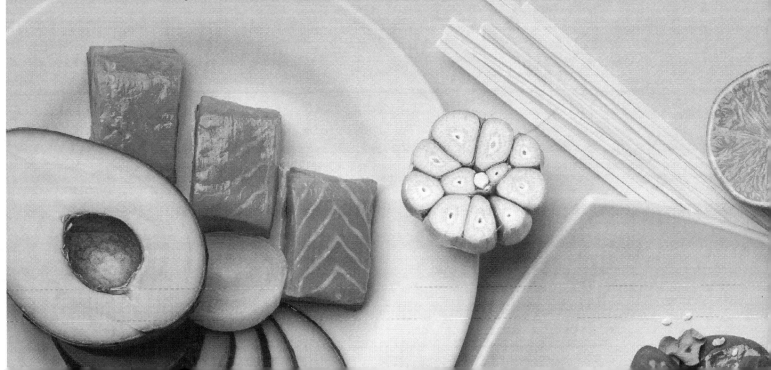

◆ Minimized Processed Food Intake

Lowering your risk of diabetes can be achieved by cutting back on your diet and focusing on consuming healthy whole foods. One easy step you can take to improve your health is to reduce your intake of processed foods, which can cause all kinds of health problems including heart disease, obesity, and diabetes. To lower your risk for diabetes, you can try cutting back on fatty foods, increasing your intake of whole grains, and taking supplements. Including fruits, vegetables, berries, and other food crops in your diet can also be beneficial in reducing your risk for diabetes.

◆ Eat High Fiber Diet

Incorporating fiber-rich foods into your diet can significantly reduce your chances of developing diabetes. This is because fiber helps to regulate blood sugar and insulin levels, while also promoting healthy digestion and weight management. There are two types of fiber: soluble and insoluble. Soluble fiber can dissolve in water, while insoluble fiber cannot.

◆ Intake of Vitamin D

Maintaining a diet that is rich in vitamin D or taking supplements can help reduce the risk of developing diabetes by improving your vitamin D levels. Vitamin D plays a crucial role in managing diabetes. Studies suggest that inadequate vitamin D intake or low blood levels of vitamin D can increase the chances of developing different types of diabetes. When the body lacks vitamin D, it can lead to malnourishment, which can affect the functioning of insulin-producing cells, increase blood sugar levels and elevate the risk of diabetes. Foods such as oily fish and cod liver oil are great sources of vitamin D. Sun exposure is also a natural way to increase vitamin D levels in the blood. However, for some individuals, it may be necessary to supplement their diet with 2,000 to 4,000 IU of vitamin D per day to maintain optimal levels.

◆ Regular Exercises

Engaging in daily physical activity, such as exercising and walking, can provide significant benefits to your body. It helps break down the sugars and fats in your body by digesting food and releasing insulin from your pancreas. Exercise also increases insulin sensitivity in the brain, which means that you need less insulin to control your blood sugar. Aerobic exercise, high-intensity exercise, and strength training can be beneficial for those who are obese and can help them lower blood sugar and control type 2 diabetes. Additionally, regular physical activity can increase insulin secretion and sensitivity, thereby preventing type 2 diabetes and lowering blood sugar levels.

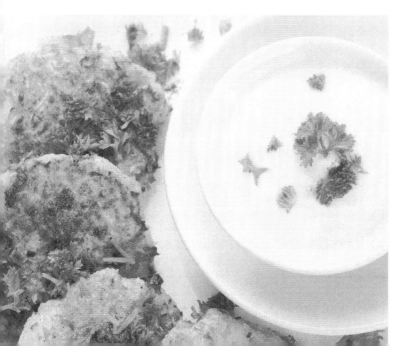

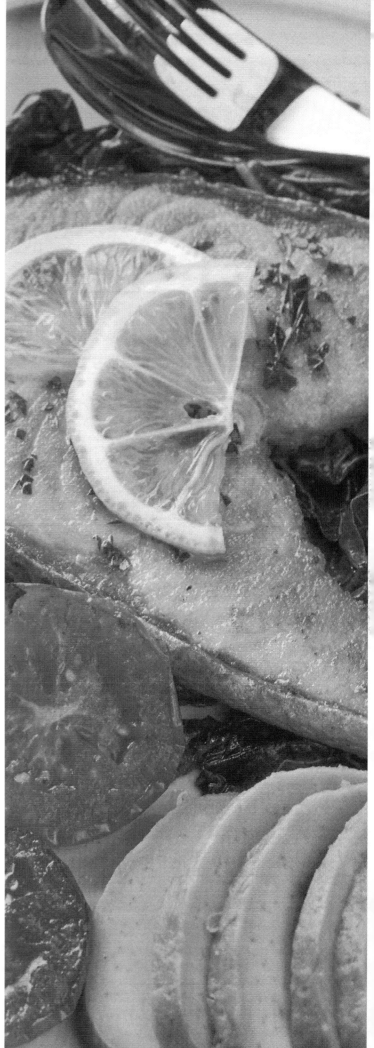

Dietary Requirements for Type-2 Diabetes

Individuals who have type-2 diabetes often experience difficulty in getting enough sugar to the brain. When the desired sugar level is not reached, the sugar in the blood increases, which can lead to problems such as damage to the kidneys, brain, eyes, and heart disease.

The best diet for individuals with type-2 diabetes includes simple carbohydrates such as brown rice, whole grains, quinoa, oatmeal, fruits, vegetables, beans, and lentils. It is recommended to avoid simple carbohydrates such as sugar, pasta, white bread, flour, cookies, and pastries. Foods that do not have a glycemic load (index) only slightly raise blood sugar levels and are a better choice for diabetics. Effective blood sugar control can help prevent the long-term problems of type-2 diabetes. Fat does not have a direct effect on blood sugar, but it can help slow down the absorption of carbohydrates.

Protein provides constant energy with little effect on blood sugar. It can help to even blood sugar levels and ease sugar cravings. Foods high in protein include beans, legumes, eggs, seafood, dairy products, soybeans, lean meats, and chicken. Diabetic "superfoods" contain chia seeds, wild salmon, cinnamon, white balsamic vinegar, and lentils. They help maintain diabetes and fulfill nutritional requirements.

A healthy diet includes lots of vegetables, a limited amount of sugar, and red meat. Dietary recommendations for individuals with type-2 diabetes include a vegetarian or vegan diet with an emphasis on exercise. Their diet should be low in glycemic load, high in vegetables, and high in vegetable fats and proteins.

Individuals with type-2 diabetes should not consume soft drinks (regularly and on a diet), refined sugars, processed carbohydrates, saturated fat, fatty junk food, high-fat foods, fruit juices high in fructose, sweets, and processed foods.

What to Eat

Maintaining a healthy diet is crucial, particularly for individuals with type 2 diabetes. There are several diets available, but it's essential to choose one that best suits your health requirements. A balanced diet for type 2 diabetes should include a diverse range of nutritious foods that provide your body with the essential fiber, vitamins, and minerals it needs to function correctly.

In addition to this, the consumption of a variety of heart-healthy oils, such as monounsaturated and polyunsaturated fatty acids, can help you maintain a healthy heart by reducing cholesterol levels. These oils can be found in sources such as nuts, seeds, avocados, and olive oil.

It's worth noting that a high fiber diet can significantly improve blood sugar control, allowing you to feel fuller for more extended periods and preventing overeating when you're not hungry. Moreover, it's crucial to choose a diet that is both safe and easy to follow while also being delicious. A diet that is too restrictive or doesn't suit your lifestyle can be challenging to manage in the long run.

Therefore, it's essential to choose a healthy diet that fits your lifestyle and tastes good. You can work with a certified dietitian to create a personalized meal plan that meets your specific dietary needs while ensuring that you enjoy the food you eat. Making healthy food choices and following a balanced diet can help individuals with type 2 diabetes manage their blood sugar levels and improve their overall health and quality of life. Here are some examples of foods you should include in your diet.

- Fruits: apples, oranges, strawberries, melons, pears, and peaches.
- Vegetables: cauliflower, cauliflower, cabbage, cucumber, pumpkin, etc.
- Whole grains: quinoa, couscous, oats, brown rice, Faro
- Beans: beans, lentils, and chickpeas

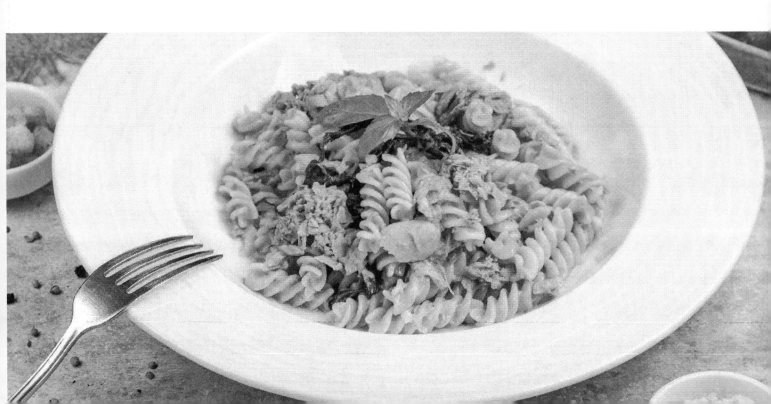

- Nuts: almonds, walnuts, pistachios, macadamia nuts, cashews
- Seeds: chia seeds, pumpkin seeds, flax seeds, hemp seeds
- Foods rich in protein: lean chicken, seafood, lean meats, beans, tempeh
- Heart-healthy fats: olive oil, avocado, canola oil, sesame oil
- Drinks: water, black coffee, unsweetened tea, soup

What to Avoid

If you have type 2 diabetes, it's important to know that there aren't any foods that you need to completely avoid. However, it's best to choose foods that are rich in vitamins and minerals while having a low fat content. By doing so, you can improve your blood sugar control and prevent the health problems associated with diabetes. Foods that are high in fiber, such as fruits, vegetables, and whole grains, are great choices as they can help regulate blood sugar levels. Additionally, lean protein sources such as chicken or fish, along with low-fat dairy products, are other healthy options to consider. On the other hand, it's recommended that you limit your intake of foods that are high in saturated fats, added sugars, and salt. These foods include processed snacks, sugary drinks, fried foods, and high-fat meats. By being mindful of your food choices and making healthier choices, you can help manage your diabetes and improve your overall health. Here are some of the foods you should limit or avoid in your diet with type-2 diabetes:

- Fatty meats: beef, lamb, chicken, black chicken
- Fatty foods: whole milk, butter, cheese, sour cream
- Sweets: candies, cookies, toast, ice cream, candies
- Non-alcoholic drinks: non-alcoholic drinks, tea sweeteners, processed juices
- Sweeteners: sugar, brown sugar, honey, maple syrup, molasses
- Processed foods: chips, microwave popcorn, processed meats, ready meals
- Fatty foods: short vegetables, fried foods, dairy-free coffee, semi-hydrogenated fats

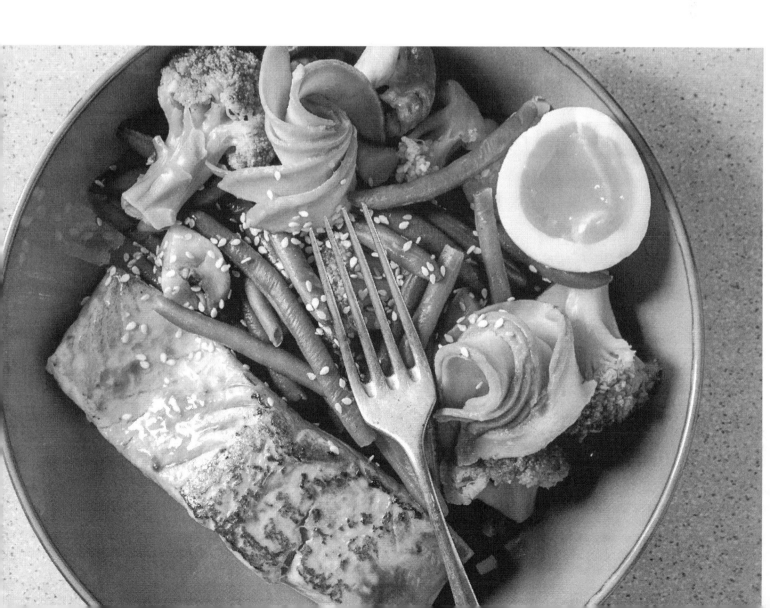

4-Week Meal Plan

Week 1

Day 1:
Breakfast: Cheese Vegetable Omelet
Lunch: Mashed Potatoes & Cauliflower
Dinner: Baked Quinoa and Tilapia
Dessert: Coconut Oats Cookies

Day 2:
Breakfast: Easy Fruit Smoothie
Lunch: Delicious Cheese Chicken Spinach Sandwiches
Dinner: Almond Chicken Satay with Peach Salad
Dessert: Strawberry Yogurt Pops

Day 3:
Breakfast: Buttermilk Pancakes
Lunch: Garlicky Black-Eyed Peas & Kale Salad
Dinner: Delicious Round Steak and Celery
Dessert: Minty Hot Chocolate

Day 4:
Breakfast: Overnight Apricot Oatmeal
Lunch: Broccoli and Rice Pilaf
Dinner: Cheese Salmon Mushroom Casserole
Dessert: Peanut Butter Energy Balls

Day 5:
Breakfast: Breakfast Walnuts Berry Quinoa
Lunch: Quinoa Pulao
Dinner: Herbs Roasted Whole Chicken with Vegetables
Dessert: Homemade Omega-3 Crackers

Day 6:
Breakfast: Cloud Eggs on Toast
Lunch: Parmesan Broccoli Millet Casserole
Dinner: Soy Beef Steak Stew
Dessert: Keto Bread

Day 7:
Breakfast: Lemon Poppy Seeds Muffins
Lunch: Cheese Quinoa Spinach Fritters
Dinner: Flavorful Crab Cakes
Dessert: Chocolate Avocado Mousse

Week 2

Day 1:
Breakfast: Egg and Ham Breakfast "Burritos"
Lunch: Wheat Berry Tabbouleh Salad
Dinner: Baked Lemon Trout with Potato Hash Browns
Dessert: Butter Pecan Cookies

Day 2:
Breakfast: Cream Cheese Blueberry Crêpes
Lunch: Baked Mac and Cheese with Vegetables
Dinner: Turkey Meatballs with Chickpea Pasta
Dessert: Raspberry-Chocolate Chia Pudding

Day 3:
Breakfast: Sweet Potato-Onion Pancakes
Lunch: Roasted Tomatoes and Cheese Sandwich
Dinner: Meat and Tomato Stew
Dessert: Lemon Avocado Dressing

Day 4:
Breakfast: Cheesy Breakfast Mushroom Casserole
Lunch: Sweet Beans Soup
Dinner: Herbed Shrimp and Ham Jambalaya
Dessert: Cherry Chocolate Cashews Milkshake

Day 5:
Breakfast: Fresh Fruit and Yogurt Smoothie
Lunch: Spicy Beans and Corn Casserole
Dinner: Crispy Chicken Thighs with Collard Greens
Dessert: Lime Beetroot Hummus

Day 6:
Breakfast: Breakfast Sausage Zucchini Hash Browns
Lunch: Beans and Bacon Stew
Dinner: Beef, Potato and Vegetables Stew
Dessert: Chocolate Cashew Raisins Truffles

Day 7:
Breakfast: Cheese Spinach Shakshuka
Lunch: Spicy Chickpea Balls
Dinner: Pesto Salmon with Asparagus
Dessert: Soft Banana Cashew Ice Cream

Week 3

Day 1:
Breakfast: Black Bean Huevos Rancheros
Lunch: Easy Zucchini Patties
Dinner: Baked Halibut and Beans
Dessert: Nutty Cranberry Cereal Mix

Day 2:
Breakfast: Tofu and Fruit Smoothie
Lunch: Flavorful Chicken and Grape Sandwiches
Dinner: Yummy Chicken and Shrimp Jambalaya
Dessert: Nuts Date Bars

Day 3:
Breakfast: Almond Butter Pancakes
Lunch: Radish and Egg Salad Sandwiches
Dinner: Easy Chuck Roast and Veggies Stew
Dessert: Cheese Garlic Kale Chips

Day 4:
Breakfast: Cheesy Brussels Sprouts with Bacon & Eggs
Lunch: Banana Peanut Butter "Sushi"
Dinner: Spicy Garlic Shrimp
Dessert: Lime-Chili Popcorn

Day 5:
Breakfast: Lemon Sausage with Eggs and Veggies
Lunch: Chickpea Pasta with Mushroom
Dinner: Cheesy Rice & Chicken Stuffed Bell Peppers
Dessert: Rosemary Nuts Mix

Day 6:
Breakfast: Sausage and Mushroom Frittata
Lunch: Vegetables Tortilla Pizza
Dinner: Juicy Steak and Mushroom
Dessert: Peanut Butter Flaxseed Balls

Day 7:
Breakfast: Pineapple & Aloe Vera Green Tea Drink
Lunch: Herbed Potatoes and Onion
Dinner: Cumin Turkey Stuffed Sweet Potatoes
Dessert: Peanut Butter Energy Balls

Week 4

Day 1:
Breakfast: Herbed Walnut Omelet
Lunch: Sweet & Spicy Chickpeas & Arugula Tacos
Dinner: Lime Coconut White Fish with Broccoli
Dessert: Coconut Oats Cookies

Day 2:
Breakfast: Avocado, Beets and Berries Smoothie
Lunch: Black Beans Tortillas with Guacamole
Dinner: Cheese Turkey Zucchini Spaghetti
Dessert: Minty Hot Chocolate

Day 3:
Breakfast: Tasty Millet Porridge
Lunch: Roasted Cauliflower Steaks with Honey Mustard Dressing
Dinner: Traditional Stroganoff Steak
Dessert: Strawberry Yogurt Pops

Day 4:
Breakfast: Raspberry and Yogurt Parfait
Lunch: Veggie and Egg Salad
Dinner: Sweet & Spicy Shrimp Skewers
Dessert: Homemade Omega-3 Crackers

Day 5:
Breakfast: Creamy Quinoa with Almonds & Blueberries
Lunch: Roasted Vegetables
Dinner: Teriyaki Chicken with Broccoli & Cauliflower Rice
Dessert: Chocolate Avocado Mousse

Day 6:
Breakfast: Homemade Summer Vegetables Quiche
Lunch: Sautéed Eggplant and Zucchini
Dinner: Roasted Rump and Vegetables Stew
Dessert: Raspberry-Chocolate Chia Pudding

Day 7:
Breakfast: Breakfast Egg Tostadas
Lunch: Cheesy Mushroom and Cauliflower
Dinner: Homemade Pot Roast and Vegetables Stew
Dessert: Chocolate Cashew Raisins Truffles

Chapter 1 Breakfast Recipes

Buttermilk Pancakes

Prep time: 10 minutes | Cook time: 10 minutes | Serves: 2

1 cup almond flour
2 tablespoons nonfat buttermilk powder
¼ teaspoon baking soda

½ teaspoon low-salt baking powder
1 cup water

1. In a bowl, blend all the ingredients, adding more water if necessary to get batter consistency desired. 2. Pour ¼ of batter into a medium nonstick skillet or a skillet treated with nonstick cooking spray. Cook until bubbles appear on the top half of pancake over medium heat. Flip and continue cooking until the center of the pancake is done, about 1–2 minutes each side. Repeat process with remaining batter.

Per Serving: Calories 143; Total Fat 2g; Saturated Fat 1g; Sodium 111mg; Carbs 26g; Fiber 1g; Sugar 4g; Protein 6g

Sweet Potato-Onion Pancakes

Prep time: 10 minutes | Cook time: 15 minutes | Serves: 4

2 medium sweet potatoes
¼ cup onions, grated
1 egg
3 tablespoons whole-wheat pastry flour

½ teaspoon cinnamon
½ teaspoon baking powder
½ cup egg whites
2 tablespoons canola oil

1. Scrub sweet potatoes; pierce skins with fork and microwave on high for 4–5 minutes. Scoop sweet potato out of skins; lightly mash with fork. 2. In a medium bowl, mix together the sweet potatoes, grated onion, and egg. Add in flour, cinnamon, and baking powder. 3. In separate small bowl, beat the egg whites until rounded peaks are formed. Gently fold egg whites into potato mixture. 4. Heat the oil until hot. Spoon batter onto skillet to form pancakes approximately 4" in diameter. Brown on both sides, about 3–4 minutes. 5. Serve hot with some unsweetened apple sauce.

Per Serving: Calories 168; Total Fat 7g; Saturated Fat 1g; Sodium 139mg; Carbs 25.87g; Fiber 3g; Sugar 3g; Protein 6g

Cheese Vegetable Omelet

Prep time: 15 minutes | Cook time: 20 minutes | Serves: 2

2 teaspoons olive oil
1 cup diced zucchini
¼ cup diced red pepper
1 cup plum tomatoes, skinned and cubed

⅛ teaspoon pepper
4 eggs
1 tablespoon Parmesan cheese
1 teaspoon minced fresh basil

1. Heat the oil and add zucchini and red pepper and sauté for 5 minutes in a non-stick skillet. 2. Add tomatoes and pepper and cook uncovered for another 10 minutes, allowing fluid from tomatoes to cook down. 3. In a bowl, whisk the eggs, Parmesan cheese, and fresh basil; pour over the vegetables in skillet. 4. Cook over low heat until browned, approximately 10 minutes on each side.

Per Serving: Calories 253; Total Fat 17g; Saturated Fat 5g; Sodium 221mg; Carbs 7g; Fiber 2g; Sugar 1g; Protein 17g

Easy Fruit Smoothie

Prep time: 5 minutes | Cook time: 0 minutes | Serves: 1

1 cup skim milk
1 cup diced mixed fruit like berries, apple, or banana
1 tablespoon honey

4 teaspoons toasted wheat germ
6 large ice cubes

1. Blend all ingredients until thick and smooth. Serve.
Per Serving: Calories 228; Total Fat 0.5g; Saturated Fat 0.1g; Sodium 308mg; Carbs 34g; Fiber 0.4g; Sugar 33g; Protein 21.6g

Fresh Fruit and Yogurt Smoothie

Prep time: 5 minutes | Cook time: 0 minutes | Serves: 2

1 cup plain low-fat yogurt
½ cup sliced strawberries
½ cup orange juice

½ cup nectarines, peeled and sliced
2 tablespoons ground flax seed

1. Blend all ingredients until thick and smooth.
Per Serving: Calories 149; Total Fat 1g; Saturated Fat 0g; Sodium 96mg; Carbs 26g; Fiber 2g; Sugar 6g; Protein 10g

Tofu and Fruit Smoothie

Prep time: 10 minutes | Cook time: 0 minutes | Serves: 1

1⅓ cups frozen unsweetened strawberries
½ banana

½ cup (4 ounces) silken tofu

1. Blend all ingredients until thick and smooth. Add a little chilled water for thinner smoothies if desired.
Per Serving: Calories 319; Total Fat 11g; Saturated Fat 2g; Sodium 19mg; Carbs 35g; Fiber 8g; Sugar 4g; Protein 20g

Overnight Apricot Oatmeal

Prep time: 15 minutes | Cook time: 0 minutes | Serves: 4

1 cup steel-cut oats
14 dried apricot halves
1 dried fig

2 tablespoons golden raisins
4 cups water
½ cup coconut cream

1. Add all ingredients in a slow cooker with a ceramic interior. 2. Set to low heat. Cover and cook overnight (8–9 hours).
Per Serving: Calories 221; Total Fat 3g; Saturated Fat 1g; Sodium 25mg; Carbs 42g; Fiber 6g; Sugar 3g; Protein 9g

Cloud Eggs on Toast

Prep time: 10 minutes | Cook time: 10 minutes | Serves: 1

2 egg whites
½ teaspoon sugar
1 cup water

1 tablespoon frozen apple juice concentrate
1 slice reduced-calorie oat-bran bread, lightly toasted

1. In a copper bowl, beat the egg whites until thickened. Add sugar in and beat until stiff peaks form. 2. In a small saucepan, heat water and apple juice over medium heat until it just begins to boil. Reduce heat and allow mixture to simmer. 3. Drop egg whites by teaspoon full into the simmering water. Simmer for 3 minutes; turn over and simmer for an additional 3 minutes. 4. Ladle "clouds" over bread and serve immediately.

Per Serving: Calories 57; Total Fat 1g; Saturated Fat 0g; Sodium 101mg; Carbs 9g; Fiber 0g; Sugar 3g; Protein 4g

Breakfast Walnuts Berry Quinoa

Prep time: 10 minutes | Cook time: 25 minutes | Serves: 4

1 cup quinoa
2 cups water
¼ cup walnuts

1 teaspoon cinnamon
2 cups berries

1. Rinse the quinoa before cooking. Place the quinoa, water, walnuts, and cinnamon in a 1½-quart saucepan and bring to a boil. 2. Lower the heat; cover and cook for 15 minutes, or until all water has been absorbed. 3. Add the berries and serve with milk, soy milk, or sweetener if desired.

Per Serving: Calories 228; Total Fat 5g; Saturated Fat 0g; Sodium 2mg; Carbs 41g; Fiber 5g; Sugar 3g; Protein 7g

Pork Loin Noodle Soup

Prep Time: 5 minutes | Cook Time: 20 minutes |Serves: 4

1 tablespoon sesame oil
2 cups sliced portobello or shiitake mushrooms
1 teaspoon garlic powder
½ teaspoon ground ginger
6 cups low-sodium beef broth
1 cup water
2 teaspoons low-sodium soy sauce

2 teaspoons rice vinegar
½ teaspoon fish sauce
2 sheets snack-size nori
2 cups packaged zucchini noodles (zoodles)
1 pound Roasted Pork Loin
¼ cup chopped scallions (optional)

1. A large stockpot should be heated to medium. Pour sesame oil into a heated pan, then add the mushrooms, ginger, and garlic powder. While intermittently stirring, cook for 5 minutes. 2. Add the soy sauce, rice vinegar, and fish sauce after adding the broth and water. Bring the broth to a boil by turning up the heat to high. 3. Strip the nori into ¼-inch pieces. 4. Add the noodles and nori to the broth when it starts to boil, and simmer for three minutes. 5. Pork loin should be cut into 8 equal pieces. Place two slices of pork loin and one tablespoon of finely chopped scallions on top of each bowl after dividing the soup among four bowls (if using).

Per Serving: Calories 660; Total Fat 28g; Saturated Fat 12g; Sodium 795mg; Carbs 51g; Fiber 2g; Sugar 5g; Protein 56g

Cheese Spinach Shakshuka

Prep time: 5 minutes | Cook time: 20 minutes | Serves: 4

1 (24-ounce) jar no-sugar-added marinara sauce, such as Rao's
¼ cup extra-virgin olive oil
½ to 1 teaspoon crushed red pepper flakes

6 ounces frozen spinach, thawed and drained of excess liquid (about 11/2 cups)
4 large eggs
4 ounces shredded mozzarella cheese

1. In a medium, deep skillet with a lid, combine the marinara sauce, olive oil, red pepper flakes to taste (if using), and spinach, and stir until well combined. 2. Bring the mixture to a boil over medium-high heat. Reduce the heat to low, cover, and simmer for 2 to 3 minutes. 3. Uncover the skillet and gently crack each egg into the simmering sauce, allowing the egg to create a crater and being careful not to let the eggs touch. Return the lid and cook, poaching the eggs until the yolks are just set, 8 to 10 minutes. 4. Uncover and sprinkle with the cheese. Cook for 3 minutes until the cheese is melted and the eggs are fully cooked, another 3 to 5 minutes. Serve warm.

Per Serving: Calories 395; Total Fat 32g; Saturated Fat 8g; Sodium 825mg; Carbs 9g; Fiber 3g; Sugar 0g; Protein 17g

Almond Butter Pancakes

Prep time: 5 minutes | Cook time: 15 minutes | Serves: 4

½ cup creamy almond butter (unsweetened)
2 large eggs
½ cup unsweetened almond milk

1 cup almond flour
1 teaspoon baking powder
Cooking spray, coconut oil, or butter

1. In a bowl, whisk the almond butter, eggs, and almond milk until smooth and creamy. Add in the almond flour with baking powder until smooth. If the batter is very thick, add additional almond milk 1 tablespoon at a time until pourable. 2. Heat a nonstick skillet and drizzle oil. Pour ¼ cup of the batter onto the hot skillet and cook for 4 to 5 minutes, until the edges begin to firm up. Flip the pancake and cook for 2 to 3 minutes on the second side. 3. You should get about 8 pancakes. Serve warm.

Per Serving: Calories 396; Total Fat 34g; Saturated Fat 3g; Sodium 180mg; Carbs 6g; Fiber 6g; Sugar 0g; Protein 16g

Black Bean Huevos Rancheros

Prep Time: 5 minutes | Cook Time: 10 minutes | Serves: 4

1 cup low-sodium black beans, drained and rinsed
Avocado oil cooking spray
½ cup jarred salsa verde

8 large eggs
1 cup packaged or fresh Pico de Gallo
4 lime wedges

1. Place a small saucepan over low heat, add the black beans and salsa verde. Cover and cook for about 10 minutes, or until the beans are well heated. 2. In the meanwhile, warm a small skillet over low heat. When the frying surface is hot, spray it with cooking spray and fry or scramble the eggs as desired. 3. Top two eggs with a quarter of the black beans and pico de gallo for each serving. Add a squeeze of lime to each serving to finish.

Per Serving: Calories 207; Total Fat 9g; Saturated Fat 3g; Sodium 580mg; Carbs 22g; Fiber 5g; Sugar 6g; Protein 9g

Egg and Ham Breakfast "Burritos"

Prep time: 5 minutes | Cook time: 5 minutes | Serves: 2

4 large eggs
¼ cup jarred pesto (preferably made with olive oil)
½ teaspoon salt

¼ teaspoon freshly ground black pepper
2 tablespoons extra-virgin olive oil
4 large slices thick-cut uncured ham or turkey

1. In a bowl, whisk the eggs, pesto, salt, and pepper. 2. Heat the olive oil in a medium skillet over medium heat. Spread the egg mix in the pan, lower the heat to low, and cook, stirring often, to scramble the eggs until just set, 3 to 4 minutes. Remove them from the heat. 3. Put the ham slices on a microwave-safe plate and microwave on high for 15 seconds, or until heated through. 4. Place one-quarter of the egg mixture along one edge of each ham slice and roll like a burrito around the eggs. Secure with a toothpick if needed, and serve warm.
Per Serving: Calories 537; Total Fat 40g; Saturated Fat 8g; Sodium 2054mg; Carbs 5g; Fiber 0.4g; Sugar 0g; Protein 39g

Lemon Poppy seeds Muffins

Prep time: 15 minutes | Cook time: 18 minutes | Serves: 12

½ cup extra-virgin olive oil
½ cup sour cream
3 large eggs
1 teaspoon vanilla extract
Zest of 1 lemon

½ cup granulated sugar-free sweetener, such as Swerve
1¾ cups almond flour
1½ teaspoons baking powder
1 teaspoon xanthan gum
1½ teaspoons poppy seeds

1. Preheat the oven to 350°F. Line a 12-cup muffin tin with liners. 2. In a large bowl, whisk together the olive oil, sour cream, eggs, vanilla, lemon zest, and granulated sweetener. Add the almond flour, baking powder, xanthan gum (if using), and poppy seeds, and mix until well incorporated. 3. Divide the batter evenly to the prepared muffin cups, filling each about three-quarters full. Bake until a toothpick inserted in the center of a muffin comes out clean, 16 to 18 minutes.
Per Serving: Calories 215; Total Fat 21g; Saturated Fat 3g; Sodium 82mg; Carbs 12g; Fiber 2g; Sugar 8g; Protein 5g

Lemon Sausage with Eggs and Veggies

Prep Time: 10 minutes | Cook Time: 15 minutes |Serves: 4

Avocado oil cooking spray
1⅓ cups peeled and diced sweet potatoes
8 cups roughly chopped kale, stemmed and loosely packed (about 2 bunches)

4 links chicken or turkey breakfast sausage
4 large eggs
4 lemon wedges

1. A big skillet should be heated at medium. Spray cooking spray on the cooking surface once it is heated. Sweet potatoes should be cooked for 4 minutes, tossing halfway through. 2. Move the potatoes to one side of the skillet and lower the heat to medium-low. Put the sausage and greens in a single layer. For 3 minutes, cook with a cover. 3. To make room for the eggs, press the sausage and veggies to one side of the skillet after mixing them together. 4. When the eggs are ready, add them in. Cook for three minutes with the lid on the skillet. Add an egg and a squeeze of lemon to each of the four pieces of the sausage and veggies.
Per Serving: Calories 152; Total Fat 10g; Saturated Fat 2g; Sodium 200mg; Carbs 8g; Fiber 2g; Sugar 2g; Protein 8g

Tasty Millet Porridge

Prep Time: 5 minutes | Cook Time: 25 minutes | Serves: 2

½ cup millet
1 teaspoon avocado oil
1½ cups unsweetened almond milk
Pinch kosher salt
Pinch freshly ground black pepper
Optional Toppings

½ cup fresh or 2 tablespoons dried fruit
1 tablespoon chopped nuts or seeds
2 tablespoons shredded Parmesan cheese
Tomatoes
Sautéed mushrooms

1. The millet should be pulsed in a coffee grinder or blender until it is roughly cut in half. 2. The millet should be added to a small pot. Over medium-high heat, stir in the oil. Until the millet is slightly toasted or fragrant, stir to coat it with the oil for 2 to 3 minutes. 3. Add the salt, pepper, and almond milk. After bringing the mixture to a boil, lower the heat to a simmer and cook the millet for 15 to 20 minutes, stirring occasionally. Creamy millet is ideal. If the liquid is too much for you, let it cook for a few minutes longer. 4. If necessary, taste and adjust the seasoning. Add whatever other toppings you choose.
Per Serving: Calories 402; Total Fat 10g; Saturated Fat 1g; Sodium 228mg; Carbs 69g; Fiber 6g; Sugar 28g; Protein 9.7g

Orange, Carrot & Oats Smoothie

Prep Time: 5 minutes | Cook Time: 0 minutes | Serves: 2

2 oranges, peeled and seeded
3 medium carrots, roughly chopped
½ cup rolled oats

1 cup nonfat plain Greek yogurt
½ cup unsweetened almond milk
½ teaspoon ground cinnamon

1. Oranges, carrots, oats, yogurt, almond milk, and cinnamon should all be put in a blender. until smooth, puree. Water can be added to a smoothie to make it thinner.
Per Serving: Calories 201; Total Fat 3g; Saturated Fat 1g; Sodium 152mg; Carbs 35g; Fiber 6g; Sugar 14g; Protein 18g

Pineapple & Aloe Vera Green Tea Drink

Prep Time: 5 minutes | Cook Time: 10 minutes | Serves: 1

8 ounces unsweetened cold green tea
3 ounces aloe vera juice
1½ cups packed fresh spinach

8 ounces frozen pineapple
2 celery stalks, roughly chopped

1. Blend the spinach, pineapple, celery, green tea, and aloe vera juice together. Processing it until smooth, pausing occasionally to use a spatula to scrape down the sides. This will make sure everything runs well. 2. Serve on top of ice cubes.
Per Serving: Calories 256; Total Fat 1g; Saturated Fat 0g; Sodium 76mg; Carbs 63g; Fiber 4g; Sugar 58g; Protein 3g

Cream Cheese Blueberry Crêpes

Prep time: 15 minutes | Cook time: 15 minutes | Serves: 2

½ cup heavy (whipping) cream, very chilled
2 to 4 teaspoons granulated sugar-free sweetener, such as Swerve, divided
1 teaspoon vanilla extract, divided
½ cup fresh or frozen blueberries

2 tablespoons orange juice
2 ounces full-fat cream cheese
2 large eggs
4 teaspoons unsalted butter, divided

1. In a bowl, mix the heavy cream, 1 to 2 teaspoons of sweetener (if using), and ½ teaspoon of vanilla. Whisk vigorously until thickened and whipped. Set aside. 2. In a saucepan, heat the blueberries, water, ¼ teaspoon of vanilla, and the remaining 1 to 2 teaspoons of sweetener over medium-high heat for 5 to 6 minutes, until bubbly. Using a fork, mash the berries and whisk until smooth. 3. Put the cream cheese in a medium microwave-safe bowl, and microwave on high for 20 to 30 seconds or until warm and melted. Add the eggs and remaining vanilla and whisk until smooth. 4. Working in batches, make the crêpes. Melt little butter in a skillet over medium heat and swirl to coat the bottom of the skillet. Pour one-quarter of the batter (about 2 tablespoons) into the skillet and swirl to spread thinly and evenly. Cook for 2 minutes until just bubbly. Using a spatula, flip to cook another 30 to 60 seconds on the second side. 5. To assemble, spoon 1 tablespoon of warm berry sauce along one side of each crêpe and roll like a burrito. Serve topped with the whipped cream.
Per Serving: Calories 474; Total Fat 44g; Saturated Fat 26g; Sodium 169mg; Carbs 8g; Fiber 1g; Sugar 0g; Protein 10g

Raspberry and Yogurt Parfait

Prep Time: 5 minutes | Cook Time: 10 minutes |Serves: 2

1½ cups nonfat plain Greek yogurt
2 drops vanilla extract
1 cup raspberries

2 tablespoons unsweetened shredded coconut
2 tablespoons chopped unsalted peanuts

1. Combine the yogurt and vanilla in a small basin, then divide into two serving bowls. 2. Raspberries, coconut, and peanuts should all be placed on top of each dish.
Per Serving: Calories 318; Total Fat 9g; Saturated Fat 2g; Sodium 85mg; Carbs 40g; Fiber 5g; Sugar 33g; Protein 22.5g

Baked Grapefruit with Yogurt

Prep Time: 5 minutes | Cook Time: 10 minutes |Serves: 1

½ grapefruit
½ teaspoon honey

½ cup nonfat plain Greek yogurt
2 tablespoons granola

1. Set the broiler to high. Line a baking sheet with aluminum foil or parchment paper. 2. Place the cut-side-up grapefruit half on the prepared baking sheet. Add the honey on top, then bake the baking sheet. Depending on how near you set the grapefruit to the broiler, cook the grapefruit until amber in color, 4 to 8 minutes, watching carefully to prevent burning. Allow to gently cool. 3. Along with a ramekin or cup of Greek yogurt sprinkled with oats, serve the grapefruit.
Per Serving: Calories 260; Total Fat 10g; Saturated Fat 5g; Sodium 112mg; Carbs 24g; Fiber 1.2g; Sugar 14g; Protein 18g

Sausage and Mushroom Frittata

Prep Time: 10 minutes | Cook Time: 15 minutes |Serves: 4

Avocado oil cooking spray
1 cup roughly chopped portobello mushrooms
1 medium green bell pepper, diced
1 medium red bell pepper, diced
8 large eggs

¾ cup half-and-half
¼ cup unsweetened almond milk
6 links maple-flavored chicken or turkey breakfast sausage, cut into ¼-inch pieces

1. Turn the oven on to 375°F for preheating. 2. Heat a large, oven-safe skillet over medium-low heat. Spray cooking spray on the cooking surface once it is heated. 3. In a pan, heat the mushrooms, green bell pepper, and red bell pepper. For five minutes, cook. 4. In the meantime, combine the almond milk, half-and-half, and eggs in a medium bowl. 5. In the skillet, add the sausage and cook for two minutes. 6. Pour the egg mixture into the skillet. Transfer the pan to the oven and bake for 15 minutes, or until the center is set and spongy.
Per Serving: Calories 264; Total Fat 17g; Saturated Fat 5g; Sodium 344mg; Carbs 11g; Fiber 1g; Sugar 6g; Protein 14g

Avocado, Beets and Berries Smoothie

Prep Time: 5 minutes | Cook Time: 10 minutes |Serves: 2

1 cup unsweetened almond milk
1 avocado, peeled and pitted
1 medium beet, peeled and roughly chopped
1 cup fresh or frozen blackberries

1 cup fresh or frozen blueberries
1 tablespoon ground flaxseed
1 cup ice

1. Almond milk, avocado, beet, blackberries, blueberries, flaxseed, and ice are all added to a blender. until smooth, puree. Add water for a thinner consistency if you want it. 2. Drink right away or keep in the fridge for up to two days in an airtight container.
Per Serving: Calories 420; Total Fat 21g; Saturated Fat 5g; Sodium 63mg; Carbs 54g; Fiber 14g; Sugar 38g; Protein 8.8g

Spiced Muesli with Cherries & Nuts

Prep Time: 5 minutes | Cook Time: 10 minutes |Serves: 5

1 teaspoon ground ginger
1 teaspoon ground coriander
1 teaspoon ground cinnamon
¼ teaspoon ground cloves
Zest of 1 lemon
3 cups rolled oats

¼ cup wheat bran
¼ cup oat bran
½ cup chopped walnuts
¼ cup raw sunflower seeds
½ cup dried cherries

1. Ginger, coriander, cinnamon, cloves, lemon zest, wheat bran, oat bran, walnuts, sunflower seeds, and cherries should all be combined in a big bowl. 2. Mix well and keep in an airtight container for up to 30 days at room temperature or for up to 2 months in the refrigerated.
Per Serving: Calories 263; Total Fat 13g; Saturated Fat 2g; Sodium 5mg; Carbs 48g; Fiber 12g; Sugar 3g; Protein 14g

Creamy Quinoa with Almonds & Blueberries

Prep Time: 5 minutes | Cook Time: 20 minutes |Serves: 2

1 cup unsweetened almond milk
½ cup quinoa, rinsed
Pinch kosher salt

¼ teaspoon ground cinnamon
2 tablespoons sliced toasted almonds
1 cup fresh or frozen blueberries

1. Bring the almond milk to a simmer over medium heat in a small saucepan. 2. Cinnamon, salt, and quinoa should be added. As you come to a boil, stir often. Then, turn the heat down to low and top with a vented lid. Cook until soft for 20 minutes, stirring occasionally. Add additional almond milk or water, 2 tablespoons at a time, for a thinner consistency. 3. Get rid of the heat. If necessary, taste and adjust the seasoning. 4. Equal quantities of cooked quinoa should be divided between two bowls, and the same number of almonds and blueberries should be sprinkled on top of each meal.
Per Serving: Calories 278; Total Fat 7g; Saturated Fat 2g; Sodium 55mg; Carbs 43g; Fiber 5g; Sugar 12g; Protein 10g

Cheesy Breakfast Mushroom Casserole

Prep time: 10 minutes | Cook time: 45 minutes | Serves: 4

4 tablespoons extra-virgin olive oil, divided
1 red bell pepper, thinly sliced
4 ounces sliced baby bella or shiitake mushrooms
1 teaspoon salt, divided

½ teaspoon freshly ground black pepper, divided
8 large eggs
1 teaspoon onion powder
4 ounces goat cheese, crumbled

1. Preheat the oven to 350°F. Pour 2 tablespoons of olive oil into a medium 8-by-8-inch glass casserole dish and swirl to coat the bottom and sides. 2. Heat the remaining 2 tablespoons of olive oil in a medium skillet. Once oil is hot, cook the bell pepper and mushrooms, season with ½ teaspoon of salt and ¼ teaspoon of black pepper, until soft and tender, 5 to 8 minutes. Remove the skillet from the heat. 3. In a bowl, whisk the eggs, remaining ½ teaspoon of salt and ¼ teaspoon of black pepper, and onion powder until well blended. Add the cooked peppers and mushrooms and goat cheese, and stir to combine. 4. Transfer the egg mixture to the prepared casserole dish and bake until set, 30 to 35 minutes.
Per Serving: Calories 374; Total Fat 30g; Saturated Fat 9g; Sodium 804mg; Carbs 4g; Fiber 1g; Sugar 0g; Protein 19g

Cheesy Brussels Sprouts with Bacon & Eggs

Prep Time: 5 minutes | Cook Time: 15 minutes |Serves: 4

Avocado oil cooking spray
4 slices low-sodium turkey bacon
20 Brussels sprouts, halved lengthwise

8 large eggs
¼ cup crumbled feta, for garnish

1. A big skillet should be heated at medium. When the surface is heated, spray it with cooking spray and fry the bacon until it is done to your preference. 2. Remove the bacon from the pan with care, then place it on a platter covered with paper towels to cool and drain. 3. Cook the Brussels sprouts for 3 minutes with the cut side down in the skillet. 4. Medium-low heat should be used. Brussels sprouts are flipped over, moved to one side of the skillet, and covered. three more minutes of cooking. 5. Uncover. Along with the Brussels sprouts, cook the eggs to your preferred doneness, preferably over medium. 6. When the bacon has cooled, crumble it. 7. Divide the Brussels sprouts into 4 parts. Place 2 eggs and a quarter of the crumbled bacon on top of each portion. Add 1 tablespoon of feta to each portion.
Per Serving: Calories 281; Total Fat 21g; Saturated Fat 4.7g; Sodium 248mg; Carbs 10g; Fiber 3.2g; Sugar 2g; Protein 13g

Breakfast Egg Tostadas

Prep Time: 20 minutes | Cook Time: 5 minutes | Serves: 2

4 eggs
¼ teaspoon ground cumin
¼ teaspoon dried oregano
⅛ cup tomato paste
1½ tablespoons milk
1 tablespoon unsalted butter
2 (6-inch) baked corn tortilla shells (tostada shells)

½ cup Sweet Drop Salsa or store-bought salsa
4 radishes, thinly sliced
Optional Garnishes:
Avocado slices
Chopped fresh cilantro
Diced red onion

1. Mix the milk, cumin, oregano, tomato paste, and eggs in a medium bowl. Place aside and give 15 minutes to relax. Cook right away if you are unable to wait the 15 minutes. (If you don't wait, the eggs tend to bleed or get watery.) 2. Prepare any optional garnish ingredients you plan to use during this waiting period. 3. Melt the butter in a large nonstick pan over medium-high heat. Stir the melted butter into the skillet's bottom and sides to evenly distribute it. Pour the eggs into the skillet, cook while carefully scraping the bottom, and then fold. Continue until the eggs have solidified into juicy curds. 4. Put one tortilla shell on each of two serving plates. Top each shell with an equal portion of eggs, then top the eggs with equal portions of salsa, sliced radish, and any of the optional garnishes you choose to use.

Per Serving: Calories 506; Total Fat 25g; Saturated Fat 8g; Sodium 263mg; Carbs 44g; Fiber 6g; Sugar 33g; Protein 24g

Homemade Summer Vegetables Quiche

Prep Time: 15 minutes | Cook Time: 45 minutes | Serves: 6

¾ cup unsweetened almond milk
½ cup nonfat plain Greek yogurt
eggs
2½ tablespoons almond flour
¾ teaspoon kosher salt
½ teaspoon freshly ground black pepper
1 cup packed shredded mozzarella cheese, divided
¼ cup chopped fresh dill

2 tablespoons avocado oil
1 small onion, minced
1 medium zucchini, cut into thin rounds
1 poblano pepper, cut into small dice
1 corn on the cob, kernels separated (about ¾ cup corn)
1 garlic clove, minced
1 cup cherry tomatoes, halved

1. Preheat the oven to 375°F. 2. Mix the almond milk, yogurt, eggs, flour, salt, pepper, ¼ cup mozzarella cheese, and dill in a large basin. Place aside. 3. Oil should be heated over medium-high heat in a large cast-iron pan. Add onion and sauté for 3 to 4 minutes, or until transparent, until it starts to shimmer. Cook the poblano pepper and zucchini for 3 to 4 minutes, or until tender. Add the corn and garlic, cook for 2 to 4 minutes. 4. Over the sautéed veggies in the pan, pour the egg mixture. Place the pan in the oven and bake for 30 to 35 minutes, or until the eggs are set and thoroughly cooked. Top with the remaining ¼ cup of mozzarella and the tomatoes. 5. Remove from the oven and allow to cool slightly before slicing.

Per Serving: Calories 246; Total Fat 12g; Saturated Fat 2g; Sodium 535mg; Carbs 20g; Fiber 2g; Sugar 8g; Protein 16g

Breakfast Sausage Zucchini Hash Browns

Prep time: 20 minutes | Cook time: 20 minutes | Serves: 4

½ cup shredded potato (from 1 medium yellow waxy potato or 2 small red potatoes)
1½ cups shredded zucchini (from 1 large or 2 smaller zucchini)
1 teaspoon salt

1-pound ground Italian pork sausage
¼ cup extra-virgin olive oil
1 teaspoon garlic powder
¼ teaspoon freshly ground black pepper

1. Combine the shredded potato and zucchini in a colander or on several layers of paper towels. Spread the salt to it and let sit for 10 minutes. Using another paper towel, press on the vegetables to release any excess moisture. 2. While the vegetables are draining, cook the sausage. Heat a deep skillet and cook the sausage, break up the meat and render the fat, until browned and cooked;8 to 10 minutes. Place cooked sausage to a bowl, reserving the rendered fat in the pan. 3. To the rendered fat, add the olive oil, add the drained potato and zucchini. Sprinkle with the garlic powder and pepper, and fry, without stirring, for 2 minutes. Using a spatula, stir the vegetables in the oil, continuing to fry for another 2 to 3 minutes until crispy and cooked .4. Return back the cooked sausage to the pot and fry for another 1 to 2 minutes, or until reheated. Serve warm.

Per Serving: Calories 533; Total Fat 40g; Saturated Fat 11g; Sodium 1507mg Carbs 18g; Fiber 2g; Sugar 0g; Protein 23g

Herbed Walnut Omelet

Prep Time: 10 minutes | Cook Time: 35 minutes |Serves: 4

1 bunch parsley, stems discarded, leaves chopped
1 bunch cilantro, stems discarded, leaves chopped
2 bunches scallions, green and white parts, thinly sliced
¼ cup chopped walnuts
8 eggs
2 tablespoons chopped unsweetened dried cranberries

¼ teaspoon ground turmeric
2 teaspoons almond flour
1 teaspoon baking powder
¾ teaspoon kosher salt
½ teaspoon freshly ground black pepper
2 tablespoons avocado oil

1. Combine the parsley, cilantro, scallions, and walnuts in a big bowl. Place aside. 2. Whisk the eggs, cranberries, turmeric, flour, baking powder, salt, and pepper in a medium bowl. On top of the herbs and walnuts, pour this mixture. 3. Heat the avocado oil in a medium nonstick pan over medium heat. When it starts to shimmer, add the egg mixture and spread it evenly throughout the pan with a spatula. Cook gradually for 20 to 25 minutes, or until the eggs are set, over low heat with the lid on. 4. To get the omelet to come out on the plate, invert a plate over the pan and delicately flip them both over. Slide the omelet back into the pan and cook for another 10 minutes, until browned on both sides and cooked through. 5. Transfer to a plate and slice into 8 wedges. Serve hot or cold.

Per Serving: Calories 72; Total Fat 7g; Saturated Fat 1g; Sodium 436mg; Carbs 2g; Fiber 0.2g; Sugar 1g; Protein 0.15g

Chapter 2 Vegan and Vegetarian Recipes

Herbs Roasted Vegetables

Prep time: 10 minutes | Cook time: 25 minutes | Serves: 6

8 ounces fingerling potatoes, quartered
8 ounces miniature red bell peppers, halved lengthwise and seeded
8 ounces mushrooms, sliced
1 cup cauliflower florets
1 onion, sliced

2 tablespoons extra-virgin olive oil
½ teaspoon salt
½ teaspoon freshly ground black pepper
1 tablespoon chopped fresh rosemary
1 tablespoon chopped fresh oregano
1 tablespoon chopped fresh parsley

1. Preheat the oven to 425°F. 2. In a large bowl, combine the potatoes, peppers, mushrooms, cauliflower, and onion. Drizzle the olive oil spice with salt, and pepper and toss to combine. 3. Arrange the vegetables on a baking sheet. Bake for 25 minutes, stirring once. Remove and toss with the rosemary, oregano, and parsley. Serve.
Per Serving: Calories 108; Total Fat 5g; Saturated Fat 1g; Sodium 209mg; Carbs 14g; Fiber 3g; Sugar 4g; Protein 3g

Mashed Potatoes & Cauliflower

Prep time: 10 minutes | Cook time: 10 minutes | Serves: 6

1 pound new potatoes, cut into 1-inch cubes
1 large head cauliflower
¼ cup unsweetened almond milk
1 tablespoon unsalted butter

½ teaspoon salt
¼ teaspoon freshly ground black pepper
2 tablespoons chopped fresh chives

1. Boil potatoes over medium-high heat until tender when pierced with a fork, about 10 minutes. Drain and return to the pot. 2. Meanwhile, fill another large pot with a couple of inches of water and a steaming basket. Boil water over high heat. Cook cauliflower until tender, 6 to 8 minutes. Drain and add to the pot with the potatoes. 3.Mash the potatoes and cauliflower together to the desired consistency. Add the almond milk, butter, salt, pepper, and chives and mix well. Serve hot.
Per Serving: Calories 125; Total Fat 3g; Saturated Fat 1g; Sodium 247mg; Carbs 23g; Fiber 4g; Sugar 4g; Protein 4g

Garlicky Black-Eyed Peas & Kale Salad

Prep time: 10 minutes | Cook time: 1 hour| Serves: 8

1 pound dried black-eyed peas, soaked in water overnight
1 bunch kale, stemmed, leaves cut into bite-size pieces

3 tablespoons extra-virgin olive oil
10 garlic cloves, minced
1 teaspoon salt

1. In a pot, cook the beans until are tender, 40 to 50 minutes. Drain and place to a bowl. 2. Boil water on high heat. Add the kale in it and cook until tender yet still bright green, 2 to 3 minutes. 3. Remove the kale from hot water and transfer it to the bowl with the beans. 4. Add the garlic, olive oil, and salt and mix well. Serve hot or cold.
Per Serving: Calories 251; Total Fat 6g; Saturated Fat 1g; Sodium 310mg; Carbs 37g; Fiber 7g; Sugar 4g; Protein 14g

Wheat Berry Tabbouleh Salad

Prep time: 10 minutes | Cook time: 1 hour| Serves: 6

1 cup wheat berries
3 cups water
1 cup chopped tomato
1 cup chopped cucumber
¼ cup sliced scallions

½ cup chopped fresh parsley
1 tablespoon chopped fresh mint
3 tablespoons extra-virgin olive oil
3 tablespoons freshly squeezed lemon juice
¼ teaspoon salt

1. In a small pot, combine the wheat berries and water. Cook the berries for about 60 minutes until tender. 2. In a bowl, combine the wheat berries, tomato, cucumber, scallions, parsley, and mint. Toss to combine. 3. In a bowl, Add the olive oil with lemon juice, and salt and mix. Pour over the salad and toss to combine. Serve immediately.
Per Serving: Calories 172; Total Fat 7g; Saturated Fat 1g; Sodium 103mg; Carbs 24g; Fiber 5g; Sugar 1g; Protein 5g

Broccoli and Rice Pilaf

Prep time: 10 minutes | Cook time: 1 hour 30 minutes | Serves: 8

Nonstick cooking spray
4 cups low-sodium chicken broth
¾ cup wild rice
¾ cup long-grain brown rice
¼ cup extra-virgin olive oil
1 large onion, chopped

2 carrots, peeled and chopped
½ teaspoon dried thyme
2 garlic cloves, minced
3 cups broccoli florets
1 teaspoon salt
½ teaspoon freshly ground black pepper

1. Preheat the oven to 350°F. Lightly coat a 2-quart casserole dish with nonstick cooking spray. 2. In a large pot, combine the broth, wild rice, and brown rice. Bring to a boil over high heat, then reduce the heat to medium. Cover it, cook until the rice is tender and the water is absorbed, around 45 minutes. Let stand for 10 minutes, covered. 3. In a skillet, heat the oil, add the onion, carrots, and thyme, and sauté until the onion becomes translucent, 5 to 7 minutes. Add the garlic and sauté for 1 additional minute. Remove the skillet from the heat. 4. Stir in the broccoli, rice, salt, and pepper. Place the mix to the casserole dish, cover, and bake until the broccoli is tender, about 30 minutes.
Per Serving: Calories 210; Total Fat 8g; Saturated Fat 1g; Sodium 340mg; Carbs 29g; Fiber 2g; Sugar 2g; Protein 6g

Vegetables Tortilla Pizza

Prep Time: 5 minutes | Cook Time: 10 minutes |Serves: 1

1 (8") high-fiber, low-carb flour tortilla
3 tablespoons low-sodium marinara sauce
¼ cup roasted vegetables such as onions, peppers, mushrooms

¼ cup shredded reduced-fat (2%) mozzarella cheese
¼ teaspoon dried oregano
⅛ teaspoon red pepper flakes

1. In a toaster oven or oven, cook the tortilla for about 3 minutes immediately on the rack. 2. Sauce should be spread over the tortilla and top it with the vegetables, cheese, oregano, and red pepper flakes. 3. Reposition for a further three minutes or until cheese has melted. Serve after cutting into six pieces.
Per Serving: Calories 140; Total Fat 7g; Saturated Fat 4g; Sodium 347mg; Carbs 10g; Fiber 2g; Sugar 4g; Protein 8g

Quinoa Pulao

Prep time: 10 minutes | Cook time: 30 minutes | Serves: 6

1 teaspoon organic canola oil
1 medium onion, sliced
2 garlic cloves, crushed
4 cardamom pods
1 cinnamon stick
2 whole cloves
1 dried red chili
1 leek, thinly sliced on the bias

½ red bell pepper, sliced
½ yellow bell pepper, sliced
1 cup quinoa
2 cups water
1 teaspoon coriander seeds
½ teaspoon salt
1 small zucchini, sliced

1. In a pot, cook the onion in hot over medium heat until it begins to soften, 3 to 4 minutes. Sauté the garlic for a minute. Add the cardamom pods, cinnamon stick, cloves, and chili and sauté for 1 minute. Add the leek and bell peppers and sauté for 2 minutes. 2. Add the quinoa and water. Boil it and add the coriander seeds and salt. Reduce the heat to low, cover, and simmer for 15 minutes. Add the zucchini, and continue to cook until the quinoa is tender and the liquid has evaporated, about 5 minutes. Fluff with a fork, remove the whole spices if desired, and serve.

Per Serving: Calories 146; Total Fat 3g; Saturated Fat 0g; Sodium 203mg; Carbs 26g; Fiber 4g; Sugar 2g; Protein 5g

Parmesan Broccoli Millet Casserole

Prep time: 10 minutes | Cook time: 40 minutes | Serves: 8

8 cups broccoli florets
2 tablespoons extra-virgin olive oil, divided
½ teaspoon freshly ground black pepper
Nonstick cooking spray
1½ cups millet
3 cups water

3 garlic cloves, minced
1 cup unsweetened almond milk
1 teaspoon dried thyme
¾ teaspoon salt, divided
8 ounces grated Parmesan cheese

1. Preheat the oven to 450°F. 2. In a large mixing bowl, toss the broccoli with 1 tablespoon of olive oil and the pepper. Spread out the broccoli on a large baking sheet and roast for 20 minutes, stirring once about halfway through. Remove and set aside. 3. Reduce the oven heat to 400°F. Lightly coat a 2-quart casserole dish with nonstick cooking spray. 4. While the broccoli is cooking, in a small pot, combine the millet and water. Boil water, then simmer on low. Cook until millet is tender and all the water is absorbed, about 15 minutes. Fluff with a fork. 5. In a skillet, Sauté the garlic for 1 minute in hot olive oil. Add the almond milk, thyme, and ¼ teaspoon of salt. Add the Parmesan cheese, stirring until it melts. Turn off the heat. 6. Transfer the millet to the casserole dish and toss with the remaining ½ teaspoon of salt. Fold in the broccoli, pour the cheese mixture over the casserole, and stir to combine. Bake the casserole, uncovered, until warmed through, about 15 minutes.

Per Serving: Calories 332; Total Fat 14g; Saturated Fat 6g; Sodium 561mg; Carbs 35g; Fiber 6g; Sugar 2g; Protein 18g

Cheese Quinoa Spinach Fritters

Prep time: 10 minutes | Cook time: 10 minutes | Serves: 5

1 cup cooked quinoa
1 large egg, beaten
¼ cup shredded nonfat mozzarella cheese
¼ cup whole-wheat bread crumbs
¼ cup finely chopped spinach
2 tablespoons finely chopped yellow onion

2 tablespoons finely chopped scallion
3 fresh basil leaves, minced
1 tablespoon garlic powder
¼ teaspoon freshly ground black pepper
⅛ teaspoon salt
1 tablespoon extra-virgin olive oil

1. Mix all ingredients instead of olive oil in a bowl. 2. Heat the olive oil in a skillet and place heaping spoonfuls of the quinoa mixture into the hot skillet. Cook until browned, 3- 4 minutes each side. Serve warm.
Per Serving: Calories 142; Total Fat 6g; Saturated Fat 2g; Sodium 138mg; Carbs 15g; Fiber 2g; Sugar 1g; Protein 7g

Beans and Bacon Stew

Prep time: 20 minutes | Cook time: 5 ½ hours | Serves: 8

2 cups dried red, or pinto, beans
6 cups water
2 garlic cloves, minced

1 large tomato, peeled, seeded, and chopped
1 teaspoon salt
2 oz. bacon

1. Combine beans, water, garlic, tomato, and salt in a slow cooker. 2. Cover. Cook on high temp setting for 5 hours, stirring occasionally. When the beans are soft, drain off liquid. 3. While the beans cook, brown bacon in a skillet. Drain, reserving drippings. Crumble bacon. Add half of bacon and 1½ Tablespoon drippings to beans. Stir. 4. Mash or purée beans. Fry the mashed bean mix in the bacon drippings. Add salt to taste. 5. Serve, with the bacon.
Per Serving: Calories 171; Total Fat 4g; Saturated Fat 1.2g; Sodium 354mg; Carbs 26g; Fiber 9g; Sugar 3g; Protein 9g

Roasted Vegetables

Prep Time: 10 minutes | Cook Time: 35 minutes |Serves: 2

1 medium sweet potato
to 15 Brussels sprouts, halved
6 teaspoons extra-virgin olive oil, divided
2 cups fresh cauliflower florets

1 medium zucchini
1 red bell pepper
⅓ cup Creamy Dill Dressing

1. Preheat the oven to 425ºF. 2. The sweet potato should be peeled and cut into 2-inch chunks. 3. The sweet potato and Brussels sprouts should be combined with 2 teaspoons of oil in a big bowl, then put in a large roasting pan and cook for 10 minutes. 4. In the meantime, mix the cauliflower with 2 teaspoons of oil in a large basin. After adding the cauliflower and cooking for an additional 10 minutes, remove the roasting pan from the oven. 5. Slice the red bell pepper and zucchini into 1-inch rounds and 1-inch rounds, respectively. Combine the zucchini and pepper with the remaining 2 teaspoons of oil in a large bowl. 6. The bell pepper and zucchini should be added after taking the roasting pan out of the oven. 15 minutes more of roasting is required. Divide the vegetables into two portions, and top with the dill dressing.
Per Serving: Calories 196; Total Fat 7g; Saturated Fat 1g; Sodium 200mg; Carbs 32g; Fiber 9g; Sugar 10g; Protein 7.6g

Mashed Cauliflower

Prep Time: 5 minutes | Cook Time: 10 minutes |Serves: 4

4 cups cauliflower florets
2 tablespoons olive oil
1 tablespoon chopped fresh chives

½ teaspoon kosher salt
¼ teaspoon ground black pepper

1. Cook the cauliflower for 10 minutes in a big saucepan of boiling water. Drain well, saving ¼ cup of cooking liquid. 2. Oil and the saved cooking liquid should be added to the blender or food processor along with the cauliflower. until smooth, purée. Season with salt and pepper before adding the chives. Serve.
Per Serving: Calories 124; Total Fat 7g; Saturated Fat 1g; Sodium 366mg; Carbs 12g; Fiber 5g; Sugar 5g; Protein 4.8g

Spicy Beans and Corn Casserole

Prep time: 15 minutes | Cook time: 6 hours| Serves: 12

15-oz. can tomato purée
1 medium onion, chopped
2 cloves garlic, chopped
1 tablespoon chili powder
1 tablespoon dried oregano
1 tablespoon ground cumin
1 tablespoon dried parsley

1-2 teaspoons hot sauce, to taste
15-oz. can black beans, drained and rinsed
15-oz. can kidney beans, drained and rinsed
15-oz. can garbanzo beans, drained and rinsed
2 15-oz. cans vegetarian baked beans
15-oz. can whole-kernel corn

1. Place tomato purée, onion, garlic, and seasonings in slow cooker. Stir together well. 2. Add each can of beans, stirring well after each addition. Stir in corn.3. Cover and cook on low 6 hours.
Per Serving: Calories 220; Total Fat 2g; Saturated Fat 0g; Sodium 270mg; Carbs 41g; Fiber 11g; Sugar 8g; Protein 12g

Sweet Beans Soup

Prep time: 20 minutes | Cook time: 14-16 hours| Serves: 8

1 lb. dried Great Northern, pea, or navy beans
2 oz. salt pork, sliced
1 qt. water
1 teaspoon salt
1 tablespoon brown sugar

½ cup molasses
½ teaspoon dry mustard
½ teaspoon baking soda
1 onion, coarsely chopped
5 cups water

1. Wash beans and remove any stones or shriveled beans. 2. Meanwhile, simmer salt pork in 1 quart water in a saucepan for 10 minutes. Drain. Do not reserve liquid. 3. Mix all ingredients in a slow cooker. 4. Cook on high until contents come to boil. Turn to low. Cook 14-16 hours, or until beans are tender.
Per Serving: Calories 269; Total Fat 5g; Saturated Fat 1.6g; Sodium 444mg; Carbs 47g; Fiber 10g; Sugar 18g; Protein 12g

Spicy Chickpea Balls

Prep Time: 5 minutes | Cook Time: 25 minutes |Serves: 4

1 (15-ounce) can low-sodium chickpeas, drained and rinsed

¼ medium onion, peeled and chopped (about ¼ cup)

1 large clove garlic, peeled

3 tablespoons chopped fresh parsley

½ teaspoon ground cumin

⅛ teaspoon ground cayenne pepper

½ teaspoon kosher salt

¼ teaspoon ground black pepper

1½ tablespoons crushed high-fiber cereal, such as Fiber One

¾ teaspoon baking powder

1. Add the chickpeas, onion, garlic, parsley, cumin, cayenne, salt, and black pepper to a food processor. Blend until the mixture is coarse and uniform, scraping down the sides as necessary. Transfer the mixture to a medium bowl. 2. Add cereal and baking powder to the bowl. Cover and chill about an hour. 3. Set the oven to 400°F. Apply nonstick cooking spray to a medium baking sheet. 4. Create twelve balls out of the mixture, then set on baking sheet. Spray some nonstick cooking spray on the balls' tops. 5. Turn balls over and cover the other side with nonstick cooking spray after baking them for 12 minutes. Bake 12 more minutes. Serve.

Per Serving: Calories 108; Total Fat 2g; Saturated Fat 0g; Sodium 443mg; Carbs 17g; Fiber 5g; Sugar 3g; Protein 5.8g

Banana Peanut Butter "Sushi"

Prep Time: 5 minutes | Cook Time: 5 minutes |Serves: 1

3 tablespoons powdered peanut butter

1 tablespoon water

1 high protein, high-fiber flatbread (approximately 100

calories)

1 medium ripe banana, peeled

¼ teaspoon ground cinnamon

1. Add water by the ¼ teaspoon to the powdered peanut butter mixture in a small bowl while swirling to achieve the required consistency. 2. Leaving about 1 teaspoon aside, spread peanut butter along the center of the flatbread. 3. Spread banana over peanut butter, then wrap up the flatbread. To seal the flatbread's edge, spread the final spoonful of peanut butter there. 4. Cut into pieces that resemble sushi rolls. Sprinkle with cinnamon and serve.

Per Serving: Calories 346; Total Fat 10g; Saturated Fat 3g; Sodium 723mg; Carbs 40g; Fiber 5g; Sugar 25g; Protein 5g

Chickpea Pasta with Mushroom

Prep Time: 5 minutes | Cook Time: 15 minutes |Serves: 4

8 ounces dry chickpea spaghetti

8 ounces white mushrooms, thinly sliced

2 cups frozen meatless crumbles

3 cups low-sodium marinara sauce

¼ teaspoon garlic powder

⅛ teaspoon ground black pepper

⅛ teaspoon red pepper flakes

1. Bring water to a boil in a saucepan, then cook spaghetti as directed on the box. 2. Over medium-high heat, warm a sizable saucepan that has been doused with olive oil spray. Add the mushrooms and cook them for 2-3 minutes. 3. After adding the meatless crumbles, heat them for 4-5 minutes, letting them brown and the water cook out. 4. Add the sauce, black pepper, red pepper flakes, garlic powder, and so on. For two minutes, stir and heat. 5. To serve, add 1 cup pasta and 1 cup sauce to each of four medium bowls and serve.

Per Serving: Calories 326; Total Fat 4g; Saturated Fat 0.5g; Sodium 63mg; Carbs 62g; Fiber 6g; Sugar 13g; Protein 11g

Baked Mac and Cheese with Vegetables

Prep time: 10 minutes | Cook time: 1 hour | Serves: 8

Nonstick cooking spray
1½ cups whole-wheat elbow noodles
4 cups frozen broccoli and cauliflower mix, thawed in a colander
1 cup shredded sharp Cheddar cheese, divided
2 large eggs, beaten

2 cups unsweetened almond milk
1 teaspoon onion powder
½ teaspoon mustard powder
½ teaspoon salt
½ teaspoon freshly ground black pepper

1. Preheat the oven to 350°F. Grease a 9-inch square baking dish with nonstick cooking spray. 2. Boil water over high heat. Cook the noodles until just tender. Drain. 3. Squeeze any excess moisture from the cauliflower and broccoli and transfer them to the baking dish. Add the noodles and the vegetables and toss them together. Add ¾ cup of cheese and toss to combine. 4. In a bowl, whisk the eggs, almond milk, onion powder, mustard powder, salt, and pepper. Pour egg mix over the noodles and vegetables evenly, and top with the remaining ¼ cup of cheese. 5. Cover and bake for about 40 minutes. Uncover it and bake again until the top is browned, another 5 to 10 minutes. Let rest for 10 minutes before serving.
Per Serving: Calories 176; Total Fat 7g; Saturated Fat 3g; Sodium 326mg; Carbs 20g; Fiber 4g; Sugar 1g; Protein 11g

Easy Zucchini Patties

Prep Time: 10 minutes | Cook Time: 20 minutes | Serves: 4

1 medium zucchini, shredded
1 small red onion, peeled and finely diced
1 large egg white

¾ cup Homemade High-Fiber Bread Crumbs
2 teaspoons all-purpose seasoning

1. Set the oven to 400°F. Set aside after gently misting a medium baking sheet with nonstick cooking spray and lining it with nonstick aluminium foil. 2. To absorb extra liquid, gently press the shredded zucchini between two pieces of paper towel. 3. Zucchini, onion, egg white, homemade high-fiber bread crumbs, and all-purpose spice are combined in a big basin. Mix thoroughly. Place mixture on baking sheet after forming it into four patties. 4. Bake for 10 minutes with baking sheet on middle rack of oven. Then, place the patties back in the oven for an additional 10 minutes of baking. 5. Remove from oven and serve immediately.
Per Serving: Calories 34; Total Fat 0.23g; Saturated Fat 0g; Sodium 47mg; Carbs 6g; Fiber 0g; Sugar 1g; Protein 1.88g

Radish and Egg Salad Sandwiches

Prep Time: 5 minutes | Cook Time: 5 minutes | Serves: 4

6 large hard-boiled eggs, diced
1 cup shredded radish
¼ cup chopped fresh cilantro
1 tablespoon olive oil
1 tablespoon unflavored rice vinegar

¼ teaspoon ground black pepper
2 cups fresh arugula
8 slices high-fiber, light whole-grain bread (40–50 calories)

1. Egg, radish, cilantro, oil, vinegar, arugula and black pepper should all be combined together in a medium bowl. 2. Divide the radish and egg salad equally among the four slices of bread to create sandwiches. Add another slice on top of each. Serve immediately.
Per Serving: Calories 373; Total Fat 15g; Saturated Fat 3.65g; Sodium 420mg; Carbs 38g; Fiber 6g; Sugar 6g; Protein 21g

Sweet & Spicy Chickpeas & Arugula Tacos

Prep Time: 10 minutes | Cook Time: 15 minutes | Serves: 6

2 (15-ounce) cans low-sodium chickpeas, drained and rinsed
¼ cup tomato paste
1 (8-ounce) can tomato sauce
1 tablespoon apple cider vinegar
1 tablespoon light brown sugar or brown sugar–style erythritol
2 teaspoons chili powder

1 tablespoon Dijon mustard
1 teaspoon onion powder
½ teaspoon garlic powder
¼ teaspoon ground black pepper
⅛ teaspoon red pepper flakes
12 hard corn taco shells
3 cups baby arugula
¼ cup chopped fresh cilantro

1. All of the ingredients—with the exception of taco shells, arugula, and cilantro—should be combined well in a medium saucepan. 2. Stirring constantly, place pan over medium heat, and simmer for 10 minutes. Get rid of the heat. 3. Arugula is added to taco shells before the bean mixture is put on top. Garnish with cilantro and serve.
Per Serving: Calories 272; Total Fat 8g; Saturated Fat 2g; Sodium 380mg; Carbs 40g; Fiber 10g; Sugar 7g; Protein 10g

Roasted Cauliflower Steaks with Honey Mustard Dressing

Prep Time: 5 minutes | Cook Time: 20 minutes | Serves: 4

For the Cauliflower:
1 head cauliflower
Avocado oil cooking spray
½ teaspoon garlic powder
4 cups arugula

For the Dressing:
1½ tablespoons honey mustard
1½ tablespoons extra-virgin olive oil
1 teaspoon freshly squeezed lemon juice

To make the cauliflower: 1. Preheat the oven to 425°F. 2. Cut the cauliflower head in half lengthwise after removing the leaves. 3. Each portion into steaks that are 1½-inches thick. 4. Garlic powder is sprinkled on both sides of each steak after frying spray has been applied to both sides. 5. On a baking sheet, cover the cauliflower steaks with foil and roast for 10 minutes. 6. To avoid the steam, take the baking sheet out of the oven and carefully draw back the foil. Steaks are flipped, then roasted for a further 10 minutes without cover. 7. Four equal servings of the cauliflower steaks should be made. Add a quarter of the arugula and dressing to the top of each serving.
To make the dressing: In a small bowl, whisk together the honey mustard, olive oil, and lemon juice.
Per Serving: Calories 54; Total Fat 2g; Saturated Fat 0.5g; Sodium 127mg; Carbs 6g; Fiber 1g; Sugar 2g; Protein 2g

Cheesy Mushroom and Cauliflower

Prep Time: 5 minutes | Cook Time: 10 minutes | Serves: 4

1 teaspoon extra-virgin olive oil
½ cup chopped portobello mushrooms
4 cups cauliflower rice

¼ cup low-sodium vegetable broth
½ cup half-and-half
1 cup shredded Parmesan cheese

1. Over medium-low heat, warm the oil in a medium skillet. When the skillet is heated, add the mushrooms and simmer for 3 minutes, turning once. 2. Add the half-and-half, broth, and cauliflower rice. stir while covering. Turn up the heat to high and boil for five minutes. 3. The cheese is added. To integrate, stir. 3 more minutes of cooking.
Per Serving: Calories 161; Total Fat 8g; Saturated Fat 4g; Sodium 532mg; Carbs 12g; Fiber 2g; Sugar 4g; Protein 10g

Black Beans Tortillas with Guacamole

Prep Time: 10 minutes | Cook Time: 15 minutes |Serves: 4

For the Guacamole:
2 small avocados pitted and peeled
1 teaspoon freshly squeezed lime juice
¼ teaspoon salt
cherry tomatoes, halved
For the Fajitas:
1 red bell pepper
1 green bell pepper

1 small white onion
Avocado oil cooking spray
1 cup canned low-sodium black beans, drained and rinsed
½ teaspoon ground cumin
¼ teaspoon chili powder
¼ teaspoon garlic powder
4 (6-inch) yellow corn tortillas

To make the guacamole: 1. With a fork, mash the avocados with the salt and lime juice in a medium basin. Add the cherry tomatoes and stir gently.To make the fajitas: 1. Slice the onion, red and green bell peppers, and bell peppers into 1-inch pieces. 2. A big skillet should be heated at medium. Spray cooking spray on the cooking surface once it is heated. The beans, onion, and peppers should be added to the skillet. 3. Stir in the garlic powder, chili powder, and cumin. Cook for 15 minutes with the lid on, stirring once. 4. After evenly distributing the fajita ingredients among the tortillas, top with guacamole and your choice of toppings.
Per Serving: Calories 234; Total Fat 15g; Saturated Fat 2g; Sodium 243mg; Carbs 22g; Fiber 11g; Sugar 2g; Protein 6g

Veggie and Egg Salad

Prep Time: 5 minutes | Cook Time: 30 minutes |Serves: 4

2 small gold potatoes, cut into 1-inch dice
4 cups fresh broccoli florets
4 cups fresh cauliflower florets
4 carrots, peeled and cut into 1-inch rounds

2 tablespoons extra-virgin olive oil
4 hardboiled eggs
⅔ cup creamy dill dressing

1. Set the oven to 450°F and raise the rack to the highest position. 2. Toss the potatoes, broccoli, cauliflower, and carrots in a large bowl with the olive oil. In one or two roasting pans, place the veggies, and roast for about 30 minutes, or until tender. 3. The eggs should be peeled and chopped. 4. Place one-fourth of the chopped eggs and dill dressing on top of each bowl after dividing the veggies among the four bowls.
Per Serving: Calories 351; Total Fat 13g; Saturated Fat 3g; Sodium 246mg; Carbs 44g; Fiber 8g; Sugar 5g; Protein 16g

Thai-Style Carrot Noodles Edamame Bowl

Prep Time: 5 minutes | Cook Time: 15 minutes |Serves: 4

2 cups frozen broccoli florets
2 cups frozen cauliflower florets
1 cup frozen shelled edamame

2 cups carrot noodles
½ cup Thai-Style Peanut Sauce

1. A big skillet should be heated at medium-high. Add the broccoli, cauliflower, edamame, and carrot noodles when they are heated, then cover. Cook for 3 to 5 minutes. 2. Remove the top and continue to cook until all water is gone. When you stir, the pan's bottom ought to be dry. 3. Separate the veggies into four equal servings and add two teaspoons of peanut sauce to each one.
Per Serving: Calories 392; Total Fat 19g; Saturated Fat 4g; Sodium 184mg; Carbs 42g; Fiber 7g; Sugar 6g; Protein 18g

Sautéed Eggplant and Zucchini

Prep Time: 10 minutes | Cook Time: 30 minutes |Serves: 4

4 tablespoons extra-virgin olive oil, divided
2 cups diced eggplant
1 cup diced zucchini
1 cup diced onion
1 cup chopped green bell pepper

1 (15-ounce) can no-salt-added diced tomatoes
1 teaspoon ground thyme
½ teaspoon garlic powder
Salt
Freshly ground black pepper

1. A large pot is warmed to medium-low. 2 tablespoons of oil should be heated before adding the eggplant and zucchini. Cook for 10 minutes while periodically stirring. As the oil will be absorbed by the eggplant, take care to avoid scorching. As required, add the final 2 tablespoons of oil. 2. Cook the onion and bell pepper for 5 minutes after adding them. 3. Cook for 15 minutes before adding the chopped tomatoes and their juices, thyme, and garlic powder. Add salt and pepper to taste.

Per Serving: Calories 101; Total Fat 6g; Saturated Fat 1g; Sodium 134mg; Carbs 11g; Fiber 4g; Sugar 6g; Protein 2g

Beans and Cauliflower on Sweet Potatoes

Prep Time: 5 minutes | Cook Time: 30 minutes |Serves: 4

4 cups fresh cauliflower florets, cut into 2-inch pieces
2 tablespoons olive oil
2 small sweet potatoes
1 cup canned low-sodium black beans, drained and

rinsed
4 lime wedges
1 cup Creamy Avocado Dressing

1. Set the oven to 425°F and raise the rack to the highest position. 2. Mix the oil and cauliflower in a large basin. Pierce each sweet potato four times with a fork. 3. On a baking pan, arrange the cauliflower and sweet potatoes. Bake for 30 minutes in the oven, or until soft. 4. Warm the beans in the microwave for up to 2 minutes during the last 5 minutes of baking. 5. Sweet potatoes should be cut lengthwise. Add the beans and cauliflower on top. Each dish should have a lime wedge squeezed over it, followed by the avocado dressing.

Per Serving: Calories 277; Total Fat 15g; Saturated Fat 2g; Sodium 637mg; Carbs 30g; Fiber 7g; Sugar 8g; Protein 7g

Cheese Chickpea Stuffed Zucchini Boats

Prep Time: 5 minutes | Cook Time: 15 minutes |Serves: 4

1 cup canned low-sodium chickpeas, drained and rinsed
1 cup no-sugar-added spaghetti sauce

2 zucchini
¼ cup shredded Parmesan cheese

1. Preheat the oven to 425°F. 2. Mix the spaghetti sauce and chickpeas in a medium basin. 3. Slice the zucchini in half lengthwise, then use a spoon to carefully scrape the seeds out of each side. 4. Add one-fourth of the Parmesan cheese on top after adding the chickpea sauce to each side of the zucchini. 5. Roast the zucchini halves for 15 minutes in the oven after placing them on a baking sheet.

Per Serving: Calories 120; Total Fat 5g; Saturated Fat 1g; Sodium 441mg; Carbs 13g; Fiber 4g; Sugar 4.3g; Protein 6.7g

Cheese Spinach Stuffed Mushrooms

Prep Time: 5 minutes | Cook Time: 20 minutes |Serves: 4

8 large portobello mushrooms
3 teaspoons extra-virgin olive oil, divided
4 cups fresh spinach

1 medium red bell pepper, diced
¼ cup crumbled feta

1. Preheat the oven to 450°F. 2. The gills should be carefully removed from the mushrooms' stems and discarded. Put two tablespoons of olive oil on the mushrooms. 3. The mushrooms should be placed cap-side down on a baking sheet and roasted for 20 minutes. 4. In the meantime, preheat a medium pan with the last teaspoon of olive oil over medium heat. When heated, stir periodically while sautéing the spinach and red bell pepper for 8 to 10 minutes. 5. From the oven, remove the mushrooms. if required, drain. Add the feta cheese after spooning the spinach and pepper mixture into the mushrooms.

Per Serving: Calories 60; Total Fat 4g; Saturated Fat 1g; Sodium 140mg; Carbs 3g; Fiber 1.2g; Sugar 1g; Protein 2.5g

Thai-Style Carrot Noodles with Cauliflower & Tofu

Prep Time: 10 minutes | Cook Time: 15 minutes |Serves: 4

Avocado oil cooking spray
4 cups carrot noodles
4 cups fresh broccoli florets
3 ounces extra-firm tofu, cut to ½-inch cubes

⅔ cup Thai-Style Peanut Sauce
½ cup chopped unsalted peanuts
¼ cup chopped scallions, for garnish (optional)

1. A big skillet should be heated slowly. Spray cooking spray on the cooking surface once it is heated. Cook the broccoli and carrot noodles in the skillet for 10 minutes with the lid on. 2. Tofu may be dried out by pressing it between sheets of paper towels in the meanwhile. Make sure the tofu doesn't crumble or break. 3. Another skillet is warmed up over medium heat. Spray cooking spray on the cooking surface once it is heated. Cooking the tofu in the skillet for 2 minutes on each side will result in golden brown tofu. 4. Add the peanut sauce and toss the veggies once they are soft. Top each part of the vegetable combination with one-quarter of the tofu after dividing the mixture into four equal sections. 5. Top with the chopped peanuts and scallions (if using).

Per Serving: Calories 713; Total Fat 41g; Saturated Fat 8g; Sodium 312mg; Carbs 67g; Fiber 5g; Sugar 8g; Protein 27g

Chickpea-Celery Lettuce Wraps

Prep Time: 10 minutes | Cook Time: 5 minutes |Serves: 4

1 (15-ounce) can low-sodium chickpeas, drained and rinsed
1 celery stalk, thinly sliced
3 tablespoons honey mustard

2 tablespoons finely chopped red onion
2 tablespoons unsalted tahini
1 tablespoon capers, undrained
12 butter lettuce leaves

1. Mash the chickpeas in a large bowl. 2. Mix thoroughly after adding the celery, honey mustard, onion, tahini, and capers. 3. Each dish should consist of three lettuce leaves overlapping on the plate, one-fourth of the chickpea mixture on top, and roll up into a wrap. Repeat with the remaining filling and lettuce leaves.

Per Serving: Calories 160; Total Fat 8g; Saturated Fat 4g; Sodium 332mg; Carbs 16g; Fiber 5g; Sugar 3g; Protein 6g

Cheesy Broccoli Bread Pudding

Prep time: 10 minutes | Cook time: 1 hour 10 minutes | Serves: 6

Nonstick cooking spray
1½ tablespoons extra-virgin olive oil
1 large onion, chopped
2 bunches Swiss chard, stemmed and leaves chopped
3 large eggs, beaten
1¼ cups unsweetened almond milk
2 tablespoons Dijon or whole-grain mustard

2 teaspoons dried sage
1 teaspoon ground nutmeg
¼ teaspoon freshly ground black pepper
5 cups chopped broccoli florets
3 slices whole-grain bread, cut into ½-inch cubes
6 ounces Cheddar cheese, cut into ½-inch cubes

1. Preheat the oven to 375°F. Lightly coat an 8-by-11-inch baking dish with nonstick cooking spray. 2. In a skillet, Add the onion in hot oil and sauté until softened, about 5 minutes. Add the chard and sauté until wilted and softened. Set aside. 3. In a bowl, whisk the eggs, almond milk, mustard, sage, nutmeg, and pepper. 4. In a bowl, toss the broccoli, bread, and cheese. Transfer half of this mixture to the prepared baking dish. Top with the chard. Add the remaining broccoli mixture to the dish. Pour the egg mix evenly over the casserole, making sure to wet all the bread pieces. 5. Bake for 1 hour, rotating the dish about halfway through. Let rest for 10 minutes before serving.

Per Serving: Calories 290; Total Fat 17g; Saturated Fat 8g; Sodium 721mg; Carbs 21g; Fiber 6g; Sugar 4g; Protein 17g

Herbed Potatoes and Onion

Prep Time: 10 minutes | Cook Time: 20 minutes | Serves: 6

4 medium potatoes, cut into ½" cubes
2 teaspoons olive oil, divided
1 medium onion, peeled and diced
1 medium red bell pepper, seeded and diced
1 tablespoon tomato paste
2 teaspoons ground sweet paprika

½ teaspoon dried thyme
½ teaspoon garlic powder
½ teaspoon ground rosemary
¼ teaspoon kosher salt
¼ teaspoon ground black pepper

1. Put the potatoes in a medium bowl that can be used in the microwave, then wrap it in plastic. Microwave 7 minutes. 2. One teaspoon of oil should be heated over medium-high heat in a medium nonstick pan while potatoes are cooking. Cook the onion and bell pepper for 7 minutes while stirring. 3. Cooked potatoes, tomato paste, paprika, thyme, garlic powder, rosemary, salt, and black pepper should all be added to the skillet. Add the final 1 teaspoon of oil in a drizzle. After combining, heat for a further 5 minutes while stirring. Serve after removing from heat.

Per Serving: Calories 222; Total Fat 2g; Saturated Fat 0.4g; Sodium 116mg; Carbs 47g; Fiber 6g; Sugar 4g; Protein 5.6g

Chapter 3 Fish and Seafood Recipes

Baked Quinoa and Tilapia

Prep time: 5 minutes | Cook time: 25 minutes | Serves: 4

1 cup quinoa, rinsed
1 cup low-sodium chicken broth
1 cup light coconut milk
1 tomato, chopped
2 teaspoons minced garlic

1 teaspoon ground turmeric
⅛ teaspoon freshly ground black pepper
1-pound tilapia fillets
2 tablespoons chopped fresh cilantro, for garnish

1. Preheat your oven at 400°F temp setting. 2. Combine the quinoa, chicken broth, coconut milk, tomato, garlic, turmeric, and pepper in a deep 9-inch square baking or casserole dish. 3. Nestle the fish in the quinoa mixture and cover the baking dish with foil. 4. Bake for about 25 minutes, until the quinoa is tender and the fish is cooked through. Top with cilantro and serve.

Per Serving: Calories 343; Total Fat 11g; Saturated Fat 6g; Sodium 86mg; Carbs 31g; Fiber 5g; Sugar 1g; Protein 31g

Cheese Salmon Mushroom Casserole

Prep time: 15 minutes | Cook time: 3-4 hours| Serves: 6

14¾-oz. can salmon, no added salt, liquid reserved
1(4-oz) can mushroom, drained
1½ cups bread crumbs
2 eggs, beaten

½ cup grated reduced-fat cheddar cheese
1 tablespoon lemon juice
1 tablespoon minced onion

1. Flake fish in bowl, removing bones. 2. Stir in remaining ingredients. Pour into lightly greased slow cooker. 3. Cover. Cook on low 3-4 hours.

Per Serving: Calories 257; Total Fat 9g; Saturated Fat 2.9g; Sodium 442mg; Carbs 21g; Fiber 1g; Sugar 2g; Protein 23g

Baked Lemon Trout with Potato Hash Browns

Prep time: 10 minutes | Cook time: 20 minutes | Serves: 4

2 large russet potatoes, chopped
¼ onion, chopped
2 teaspoons minced garlic
½ teaspoon smoked paprika
2 tablespoons olive oil, divided

Sea salt
Freshly ground black pepper
4 (4-ounce) boneless, skinless trout fillets
1 tablespoon chopped fresh parsley
1 lemon, quartered

1. Preheat the oven to 400°F. Manage a baking sheet with parchment paper. 2. In a large bowl, toss the potatoes, onion, garlic, paprika, and 1 tablespoon of the oil. Spread the potatoes on half the baking sheet and season lightly with salt and pepper. 3. Place the fish on the other half of the baking sheet, brush with 1 tablespoon of oil, and spice with salt and pepper. 4. Bake for about 20 minutes, tossing halfway through, until the potatoes are golden and lightly crispy and the fish is flaky. 5. Serve topped with parsley and lemon wedges.

Per Serving: Calories 349; Total Fat 10g; Saturated Fat 2g; Sodium 85mg; Carbs 35g; Fiber 3g; Sugar 2g; Protein 27g

Sesame Salmon with Bok Choy

Prep time: 12 minutes | Cook time: 18 minutes | Serves: 4

4 (4-ounce) salmon fillets
Sea salt
Freshly ground black pepper
4 teaspoons olive oil, divided

¼ cup maple syrup
¼ cup sesame seeds
16 baby bok choy, quartered
Juice of 1 lemon

1. Preheat the oven to 400°F. Manage a baking sheet with parchment paper and set aside. 2. Season the salmon with salt and pepper. 3. In a skillet, Pan-sear the salmon on both sides for about 3 minutes in total, turning halfway through. Place the fish on one-third of the baking sheet. Spread maple syrup on each fillet and top with sesame seeds. 4. In a large bowl, toss the bok choy with remaining 3 teaspoons of oil and lemon juice. Spice with salt and pepper and place on the remaining two-thirds of the baking sheet. 5. Bake until the fish easily flakes and the bok choy is tender-crisp, about 15 minutes. Serve.

Per Serving: Calories 329; Total Fat 17g; Saturated Fat 3g; Sodium 108mg; Carbs 19g; Fiber 5g; Sugar 12g; Protein 25g

Cajun Salmon and Vegetables Po'boy

Prep time: 20 minutes | Cook time: 10 minutes | Serves: 4

4 (4-ounce) skinless salmon fillets
2 teaspoons Cajun seasoning
2 teaspoons olive oil
1 cup finely shredded cabbage
1 large carrot, shredded

1 scallion, sliced
¼ cup low-fat plain Greek yogurt
1 tablespoon apple cider vinegar
1 teaspoon maple syrup
4 crusty whole-wheat rolls, halved

1. Preheat your oven at 400°F temp setting. 2. Season the salmon fillets with the Cajun seasoning. 3. In an ovenproof skillet, sear the salmon for 2 minutes per side, then place the skillet in the oven. Roast salmon for about 6 minutes. Place the cooked salmon in plate and set it aside. 4. In a bowl, toss the cabbage, carrot, scallion, yogurt, vinegar, and maple syrup until well combined. 5. Place a salmon fillet on each roll and top with of the cabbage mixture. Serve.

Per Serving: Calories 326; Total Fat 11g; Saturated Fat 3g; Sodium 276mg; Carbs 25g; Fiber 3g; Sugar 5g; Protein 30g

Delicious Cheesy Tomato Tuna Melts

Prep time: 5 minutes | Cook time: 5 minutes | Serves: 2

1 (5-ounce) can chunk light tuna packed in water, drained
2 tablespoons plain nonfat Greek yogurt
2 teaspoons freshly squeezed lemon juice
2 tablespoons finely chopped celery

1 tablespoon finely chopped red onion
Pinch cayenne pepper
1 large tomato, cut into ¾-inch-thick rounds
½ cup shredded cheddar cheese

1. Preheat the broiler to high. 2. In a bowl, mix the tuna, yogurt, lemon juice, celery, red onion, and cayenne pepper. Stir well. 3. Arrange the tomato on a baking sheet. Top each with some tuna salad and cheddar cheese. 4. Broil the tomatoes for 3- 4 minutes until the cheese is melted and bubbly. Serve.

Per Serving: Calories 243; Total Fat 10g; Saturated Fat 2g; Sodium 444mg; Carbs 7g; Fiber 1g; Sugar 2g; Protein 30g

Herbed Shrimp and Ham Jambalaya

Prep time: 25 minutes | Cook time: 1 ½ hours| Serves: 8

2 tablespoons margarine
2 medium onions, chopped
2 green bell peppers, chopped
3 ribs celery, chopped
1 cup chopped extra-lean, lower-sodium cooked ham
2 garlic cloves, chopped
1½ cups minute rice
1½ cups 99% fat-free, lower-sodium beef broth

1 (28-oz.) can chopped tomatoes
2 tablespoons chopped parsley
1 teaspoon dried basil
½ teaspoon dried thyme
¼ teaspoon pepper
⅛ teaspoon cayenne pepper
1 lb. shelled, deveined, medium-size shrimp
1 tablespoon chopped parsley

1. Melt margarine in slow cooker set on high. Add onions, peppers, celery, ham, and garlic. Cook 30 minutes. 2. Add rice. Cover and cook 15 minutes. 3. Add broth, tomatoes, 2 tablespoons parsley, and seasonings. Cover and cook on high temp setting for 1 hour. 4. Add shrimp. Cook on high temp setting 30 minutes, or until liquid is absorbed. 5. Garnish with parsley.

Per Serving: Calories 205; Total Fat 4g; Saturated Fat 0.8g; Sodium 529mg; Carbs 26g; Fiber 3g; Sugar 7g; Protein 16g

Baked Halibut and Beans

Prep time: 10 minutes | Cook time: 20 minutes | Serves: 4

1 (15-ounce) can low-sodium white beans, drained and rinsed
1 cup baby spinach leaves
1 cup chopped Swiss chard
12 medium tomatoes, chopped

4 (4-ounce) halibut fillets
Sea salt
Freshly ground black pepper
2 teaspoons olive oil
1 tablespoon chopped fresh basil

1. Preheat the oven to 400°F. Grease a 10-inch square baking dish with cooking spray. 2. Layer the beans, spinach, Swiss chard, and tomatoes in the bottom of the baking dish. Place the fish in the dish, season with salt and black pepper, and drizzle with the olive oil. 3. Foil cover and bake for about 20 minutes, until the fish flakes easily. 4. Serve topped with basil.

Per Serving: Calories 290; Total Fat 5g; Saturated Fat 1g; Sodium 164mg; Carbs 33g; Fiber 9g; Sugar 10g; Protein 31g

Honey-Mustard Glazed Salmon

Prep time: 5 minutes | Cook time: 20 minutes | Serves: 4

Nonstick cooking spray
2 tablespoons whole-grain mustard
1 tablespoon honey
2 garlic cloves, minced

¼ teaspoon salt
¼ teaspoon freshly ground black pepper
1-pound salmon fillet

1. Preheat your oven at 425°F. manage a baking sheet with cooking spray. 2. In a small bowl, whisk together the mustard, honey, garlic, salt, and pepper. 3. Place the fillet on the baking sheet, skin-side down. Spoon the sauce onto the salmon and spread evenly. 4. Roast it for 15-20 minutes, depending on the thickness of the fillet, until the flesh flakes easily.

Per Serving: Calories 186; Total Fat 7g; Saturated Fat 0.4g; Sodium 312mg; Carbs 6g; Fiber 0g; Sugar g; Protein 23g

Homemade Fish Tacos

Prep time: 20 minutes | Cook time: 10 minutes | Serves: 4

1 teaspoon blackening spice
4 (4-ounce) haddock fillets
1 teaspoon olive oil
1 avocado, pitted and diced
1 tomato, chopped

1 scallion, finely chopped
1 tablespoon chopped fresh cilantro
Juice of 1 lime
8 (4-inch) corn tortillas, at room temperature
1 cup finely shredded lettuce

1. Rub the blackening spice all over the fish. 2. In a skillet, Pan-sear the fish for about 10 minutes in total, turning halfway through, until just cooked through and golden. Transfer the fish to a plate and, using a fork, break the fish into large chunks. 3. In a bowl, combine the avocado, tomato, scallion, cilantro, and lime juice. 4. Divide the fish on tortillas and top with the salsa and lettuce. Fold the tortillas over and serve 2 per person.
Per Serving: Calories 259; Total Fat 10g; Saturated Fat 1g; Sodium 252mg; Carbs 23g; Fiber 6g; Sugar 2g; Protein 22g

Lemon-Herb Baked Salmon

Prep time: 5 minutes | Cook time: 20 minutes | Serves: 4

Nonstick cooking spray
½ teaspoon freshly ground black pepper
¼ teaspoon salt

Zest and juice of ½ lemon
¼ teaspoon dried thyme
1-pound salmon fillet

1. Preheat your oven at 425°F. Manage a baking sheet with cooking spray. 2. In a small bowl, combine the pepper, salt, lemon zest and juice, and thyme. Stir to combine. 3. Place the spiced salmon on the baking sheet, skin-side down. Spread the seasoning mixture evenly over the fillet. 4. Bake it for 15-20 minutes, until the flesh flakes easily.
Per Serving: Calories 163; Total Fat 7g; Saturated Fat 0.8g; Sodium 167mg; Carbs 1g; Fiber 0g; Sugar 0g; Protein 23g

Baked Salmon & Broccoli with Tamari-Ginger Sauce

Prep time: 10 minutes | Cook time: 15 minutes | Serves: 4

Nonstick cooking spray
1 tablespoon low-sodium tamari or gluten-free soy sauce
Juice of 1 lemon
1 tablespoon honey
1 (1-inch) piece fresh ginger, grated
1 garlic clove, minced

1-pound salmon fillet
¼ teaspoon salt, divided
⅛ teaspoon freshly ground black pepper
2 broccoli heads, cut into florets
1 tablespoon extra-virgin olive oil

1. Preheat the oven to 400°F. Manage a baking sheet with cooking spray. 2. In a small bowl, mix the tamari, lemon juice, honey, ginger, and garlic. Set aside. 3. Place the salmon on the baking sheet; skin-side down. Season with ⅛ teaspoon of salt and the pepper. 4. In a mixing bowl, toss the broccoli and olive oil. Season with the remaining ⅛ teaspoon of salt. Arrange in the baking sheet next to the salmon. Bake for 15 to 20 minutes until the salmon flakes easily with a fork and the broccoli is fork-tender. 5. In a pan, bring the tamari-ginger mixture to a simmer and cook for 1-2 minutes until thicken. 6.Drizzle the sauce and serve.
Per Serving: Calories 238; Total Fat 11g; Saturated Fat 0.8g; Sodium 334mg; Carbs 11g; Fiber 2g; Sugar 6g; Protein 25g

Tuna and Veggie Salad

Prep Time: 5 minutes | Cook Time: 5 minutes |Serves: 2

1 (5-ounce) can water-packed solid white tuna, drained
½ cup diced celery
¼ cup diced yellow onion
½ cup diced red bell pepper
¼ cup plain nonfat Greek yogurt

1 teaspoon Dijon mustard
1 teaspoon lemon juice
¼ teaspoon honey
2 tablespoons raisins
2 cups tightly packed mixed salad greens

1. Flake the tuna into a medium bowl using a fork. Mix thoroughly after adding the raisins, celery, yogurt, mustard, lemon juice, onion, and bell pepper. 2. Serve over salad greens.
Per Serving: Calories 177; Total Fat 4g; Saturated Fat 1g; Sodium 399mg; Carbs 13g; Fiber 5g; Sugar 5g; Protein 23g

Pesto Salmon with Asparagus

Prep Time: 10 minutes | Cook Time: 15 minutes |Serves: 2

2 (6-ounce) skin-on salmon fillets
⅛ teaspoon kosher salt
6 teaspoons canola oil, divided

¼ cup carrot top pesto, or store-bought pesto
1 bunch asparagus
1 lemon, quartered

1. Salt both fillets after thoroughly drying the fish after rinsing it. 2. 2 teaspoons of oil should be heated to a medium-high temperature in a big skillet. Carefully lay the salmon in the skillet skin-side down when it starts to shimmer. Cook the fish for 3 to 4 minutes, or until approximately one-fourth of it is opaque and the skin is crispy and golden. 3. For an additional two to three minutes, flip the salmon over. Each fillet should have half the pesto on it. 4. Salmon should be taken out of the pan and given time to rest. (The fish will keep cooking.) 5. Add the remaining oil to the skillet and place it back on the burner over medium-high heat. Add the asparagus when it starts to simmer and cook for approximately 3 minutes, turning regularly, until it is tender-crisp and just starting to brown. 6. With the salmon and lemon wedges on the side, plate the asparagus after removing it from the pan.
Per Serving: Calories 400; Total Fat 23g; Saturated Fat 3g; Sodium 823mg; Carbs 3g; Fiber 0.8g; Sugar 1g; Protein 45g

Sweet & Spicy Shrimp Skewers

Prep Time: 25 minutes | Cook Time: 5 minutes |Serves: 2

¼ cup lime juice
4 teaspoons light brown sugar
½ teaspoon chili powder

8 ounces (about 12–14) shrimp, shelled with tails remaining and deveined

1. Mix the lime juice, brown sugar, and chili powder in a small bowl. 2. Put the lime mixture and shrimp in a large plastic bag with a zip-top closure. 10 minutes of marinating on the counter. 3. Set a gas or charcoal grill to high heat in the meanwhile. Four wooden skewers should spend 10 minutes in water. 4. Take shrimp out of bag, then throw away marinade. On each skewer, thread 3 to 4 shrimp. 5. Grill shrimp for 2 minutes per side, or until just pink. Serve.
Per Serving: Calories 400; Total Fat 23g; Saturated Fat 5g; Sodium 223mg; Carbs 39g; Fiber 3.2g; Sugar 33g; Protein 14g

Refreshing Tuna and Sorghum Salad

Prep Time: 5 minutes | Cook Time: 5 minutes |Serves: 2

1 cup packed cooked whole-grain sorghum
1 (5-ounce) can water-packed no-salt-added solid
 white tuna, drained
1 cup grape tomatoes
¼ cup diced red onion
½ medium avocado, peeled, pitted, and diced
1 tablespoon olive oil

1 tablespoon plain nonfat Greek yogurt
2 tablespoons balsamic vinegar
¾ teaspoon honey
1/16 teaspoon kosher salt
1/16 teaspoon ground black pepper
2 cups romaine lettuce, chopped

1. Add sorghum, tuna, tomatoes, onion, and avocado to a medium bowl. 2. Combine oil, yogurt, vinegar, honey, salt, and black pepper in a small bowl. 3. Stir the tuna mixture with 2 tablespoons of the dressing. Serve with additional 1 teaspoon dressing drizzled over lettuce. Save any leftover dressing for another occasion.
Per Serving: Calories 564; Total Fat 19g; Saturated Fat 3g; Sodium 1223mg; Carbs 74g; Fiber 9g; Sugar 20g; Protein 28g

Spicy Garlic Shrimp

Prep Time: 5 minutes | Cook Time: 5 minutes |Serves: 4

1 tablespoon olive oil
10 medium cloves garlic, peeled and chopped
1-pound extra-large shrimp (approximately 26–30),
shelled and deveined

¼ teaspoon kosher salt
½ teaspoon ground paprika
¼ teaspoon red pepper flakes

1. Heat oil in a medium sauté pan over medium heat. Add the garlic and cook for about 30 seconds, or until fragrant but not browned. 2. Approximately 2 minutes later, add the salt and shrimp, and stir regularly until the shrimp is cooked through. 3. Turn off the heat and add the paprika. Add red pepper flakes and serve.
Per Serving: Calories 173; Total Fat 15g; Saturated Fat 2g; Sodium 981mg; Carbs 10g; Fiber 3.9g; Sugar 0.3g; Protein 1.5g

Lime Shrimp and Mixed Greens Salad

Prep Time: 15 minutes | Cook Time: 5 minutes |Serves: 2

1 cup cubed melon
1 cup diced cucumber
cups mixed greens

¼ cup Creamy Coconut and Lime Dressing
8 ounces peeled, cleaned, and cooked shrimp

1. Mix the melon, cucumber, mixed greens, and salad dressing in a medium bowl. Toss the ingredients in the dressing to coat them completely. 2. Spread half of the cooked shrimp on each platter and divide the dressed greens between them. 3. Dress only what you intend to eat if you don't intend to finish the salad right away or know you'll have leftovers. Undressed salad can be kept in the fridge for up to three days in an airtight container. Just before dining, dress the leftovers.
Per Serving: Calories 200; Total Fat 1g; Saturated Fat 1g; Sodium 275mg; Carbs 51g; Fiber 8g; Sugar 41g; Protein 4g

Paneer with Spiced Pureed Spinach

Prep Time: 15 minutes | Cook Time: 25 minutes | Serves: 4

1 tomato, roughly chopped
2 (10-ounce) packages frozen spinach, thawed and drained
1 cup chopped fresh cilantro
1 hot chile pepper, seeded and chopped (optional)
3 tablespoons avocado oil, divided
1 medium onion, minced
1 tablespoon peeled and grated fresh ginger

2 garlic cloves, minced
½ teaspoon chili powder (Indian Kashmiri, if you can find it)
2 teaspoons ground coriander
1 teaspoon ground cumin
¼ teaspoon ground turmeric
½ teaspoon kosher salt
12 ounces fresh Indian paneer cheese, cubed

1. Tomato, spinach, cilantro, and chili pepper, if used, should all be combined in a blender. until smooth, puree. 2. 1½ tablespoons of oil should be heated over medium heat in a large cast-iron pan or skillet. Add the onion to the shimmering oil and cook for 3 to 4 minutes. 3. After cooking the ginger and garlic for 2 to 3 minutes, add the salt, chili powder, coriander, cumin, and turmeric. Spices should be aromatic after 1 to 2 minutes of stirring and cooking. 4. Blend the tomato and spinach combination together with the onion until completely smooth. To taste and season as necessary. 5. The cast-iron pan should now contain the final 1 ½ tablespoons of oil. Carefully stir in the paneer after it starts to shimmer. Start by swirling to thoroughly distribute the oil over each cube, then stop and let the paneer brown for about two minutes on one side. Every two minutes, rotate each cube to ensure that at least two sides are browned. 6. Spread the cooked, seared paneer with an equal layer of the pureed spinach mixture. Stir slowly to preserve the paneer's integrity. Cook for around 3 minutes.
Per Serving: Calories 227; Total Fat 17g; Saturated Fat 2g; Sodium 591mg; Carbs 12g; Fiber 5g; Sugar 3g; Protein 9g

Flavorful Crab Cakes

Prep Time: 10 minutes | Cook Time: 20 minutes | Serves: 4

1-pound fresh lump crabmeat
¾ cup almond flour
1 large egg
2 scallions, both white and green parts, chopped
1 tablespoon grainy mustard
1 tablespoon chopped fresh parsley, or 1 teaspoon dried

1 teaspoon lemon zest
¼ teaspoon hot sauce (optional)
Sea salt
Freshly ground black pepper
Nonstick cooking spray
Lemon wedges, for serving

1. Until the mixture holds together when pushed with your hands, combine the crabmeat, almond flour, egg, scallions, mustard, parsley, lemon zest, and spicy sauce (if using) in a large bowl. 2. Create 12 patties out of the mixture, then arrange them on a platter. Refrigerate for around 30 minutes, or until firm. 3. Put a sizable skillet over medium-high heat and coat it with nonstick cooking spray. The crab cakes should be cooked for 10 minutes per side or until golden brown. Serve with lemon wedges.
Per Serving: Calories 379; Total Fat 4g; Saturated Fat 1g; Sodium 65mg; Carbs 44g; Fiber 20g; Sugar 1g; Protein 44g

Lime Coconut White Fish with Broccoli

Prep Time: 10 minutes | Cook Time: 10 minutes |Serves: 6

1-pound white fish, cut into 1¼-inch-by-4-inch pieces
Juice of 1 lime
¼ cup coconut cream
2 cups unsweetened shredded coconut
⅓ cup almond meal
1 teaspoon curry powder
½ teaspoon ground cumin

¼ teaspoon paprika
½ teaspoon kosher salt, divided
3 tablespoons avocado oil, divided
2 (10.5-ounce) bags frozen broccoli, thawed, drained, and patted dry
1 large lemon, cut into 12 wedges
1 lime, cut into 6 wedges

1. Fish, lime juice, and coconut cream should all be combined in a big dish. 15 min to 1 hour should be given for the fish to marinade. Fish should be taken out of the marinade. 2. Over medium-high heat, preheat a large frying pan or cast-iron skillet. Toasted the coconut in the skillet until golden brown, turning gently but frequently to prevent burning. Almond meal, curry powder, cumin, paprika, and ¼ teaspoon of salt are then added to the big bowl with the coconut. 3. Put a rack in the center of the oven. Set the broiler to high. Use parchment paper to cover a baking sheet. 4. Brush each piece of fish with two tablespoons of oil as the oven is heating up, and then throw it in the coconut mixture to coat it completely. Place the coconut-coated fish on the baking sheet that has been prepared. 5. On the oven rack, put the baking sheet, and bake for about three minutes. Once the fish is cooked through and the coating has browned, flip the pieces over and cook for an additional three minutes. If the outside of the fish is browned but the meat is still raw, keep it in the oven for an additional three to five minutes after turning off the oven. 6. Bring the frying pan back to the stovetop and heat it to medium-high while the fish cooks. Remaining 1 tablespoon of oil should be added. Add the remaining ¼ teaspoon of salt and the broccoli when it starts to shimmer. 7. Cook the broccoli for 3 to 5 minutes while stirring regularly, until it is hot and vibrant green. Do this in two batches if your pan is too small to fit all of the broccoli. As the broccoli is done cooking, squeeze some fresh lemon juice on top. 8. With the lime wedges and any residual lemon wedges, serve the cooked fish and sautéed broccoli.

Per Serving: Calories 210; Total Fat 12g; Saturated Fat 5g; Sodium 329mg; Carbs 10g; Fiber 3.2g; Sugar 3.3g; Protein 16g

Lemony Sardines Salad

Prep Time: 5 minutes | Cook Time: 10 minutes |Serves: 4

3 tablespoons olive oil
Juice of 1 lemon
⅛ teaspoon freshly ground black pepper
10 black olives, pitted and chopped

24 fresh sardines, butterflied
12 cups mixed greens
3 cups cherry tomatoes, halved

1. Olive oil, lemon juice, pepper, and olives should all be combined in a small bowl. Place the sardines in a plastic bag or sealable container after adding this marinade. For at least 15 minutes and up to 24 hours, seal the meat and let it marinade. 2. Over medium-high heat, preheat a cast-iron skillet, grill pan, or frying pan. The sardines should be carefully taken out of the marinade, placed skin-side down in the skillet, and cooked for 3 minutes or until golden brown. The opposite side should be cooked for 3 minutes, or until golden brown. 3. On four plates, evenly distribute the greens and tomatoes. Add 6 cooked sardines on the top of each salad.

Per Serving: Calories 343; Total Fat 19g; Saturated Fat 2g; Sodium 597mg; Carbs 22g; Fiber 6g; Sugar 14g; Protein 21g

Chapter 4 Chicken and Poultry Recipes

Almond Chicken Satay with Peach Salad

Prep time: 10 minutes | Cook time: 5 minutes | Serves: 4

For the Satay
⅔ cup ground almonds
5 garlic cloves, minced
1 teaspoon berbere or any hot pepper spice
(e.g., cayenne pepper or chili powder)
⅛ teaspoon freshly ground black pepper
¼ teaspoon kosher salt
3 tablespoons canola oil
1 tablespoon maple syrup
1½ pounds chicken breasts, boneless, skinless,

cut into ¼-inch-thick strips
½ cup water
For the Salad
Zest and juice of 1 lemon
3 tablespoons extra-virgin olive oil
1 large fennel bulb, halved, cored, and very thinly sliced
2 peaches, pitted and thinly cut into wedges
¼ cup fresh parsley leaves
To make the satay

1. In a bowl, add the almonds, garlic, berbere, black pepper, salt, canola oil, and maple syrup. Mix until thoroughly combined. Add the chicken and coat evenly. Marinate for at least 30 minutes. 2. Preheat the grill, or place an oven rack in the topmost position in the oven and preheat the broiler to high. 3. Brush away some of the marinade before threading the chicken onto skewers. Evenly distribute the chicken among the skewers. Grill it for 3 minutes on each side. 4. Scrape the leftover marinade into a saucepan, add the water, and bring it to a boil over high heat. Transfer to a small bowl to serve with the chicken skewers and salad. 5. To make the salad: Put the lemon zest with juice into a medium bowl. Slowly whisk in the olive oil. 6. Add the shaved fennel, peaches, and parsley leaves and toss gently to coat with the dressing. 7. Allow the salad to rest while you finish preparing the chicken.
Per Serving: Calories 539; Total Fat 32g; Saturated Fat 2g; Sodium 236mg; Carbs 23g; Fiber 4.5g; Sugar 13g; Protein 41g

Herbs Roasted Whole Chicken with Vegetables

Prep time: 10 minutes | Cook time: 45 minutes | Serves: 6

1 (3½- to 4-pound) whole chicken, butterflied
2½ tablespoons canola oil, divided
3 garlic cloves, minced
4 thyme sprigs, broken apart into large pieces
4 rosemary sprigs, broken apart into large pieces

½ teaspoon kosher salt
½ teaspoon freshly ground black pepper, divided
5 parsnips, cut lengthwise in ½-inch strips
1 rutabaga, cut into ½-inch cubes
1 onion, cut into 1-inch wedges

1. Preheat the oven to 450°F temp setting. 2. Using paper towels, pat dry the chicken. Carefully separate the skin from the chicken, then rub 1 tablespoon of oil between them and on the outside of the skin. Evenly disperse the minced garlic and thyme and rosemary sprigs under the skin. Season the skin on all sides with the salt and ¼ teaspoon of black pepper. Set aside while you prep the vegetables. 3. In a medium bowl, thoroughly combine the remaining 1½ tablespoons of oil and remaining ¼ teaspoon of pepper with the parsnips, rutabaga, and onion. Place the vegetables and place the chicken on top. Position the chicken breasts to be in the center of the baking sheet, skin-side up. The legs should be splayed close to the edges. Roast the chicken and veggies for 40-45 minutes. 4. Transfer the chicken to a clean, sanitized cutting board, cover it with aluminum foil, and allow it to rest for 10 minutes. 5. Meanwhile, place the vegetables on a platter or keep them warm in the oven with the heat turned off.6. Carve and serve it with the roasted vegetables.
Per Serving: Calories 514; Total Fat 25g; Saturated Fat 10g; Sodium 293mg; Carbs 33g; Fiber 8.5g; Sugar 10g; Protein 39g

Tandoori Chicken Breasts with Cauliflower Rice

Prep time: 5 minutes | Cook time: 30 minutes | Serves: 4

For the Tandoori Chicken:

4 boneless, skinless chicken breasts
4 tablespoons freshly squeezed lemon juice
¼ teaspoon kosher salt
¼ teaspoon ground turmeric
2 garlic cloves, minced
1 tablespoon chopped fresh ginger

½ teaspoon ground cardamom
¾ teaspoon ground cumin
2 teaspoons paprika
½ cup nonfat plain Greek yogurt
½ tablespoon olive oil

For the Cauliflower Rice:

1 (1½-pound) head cauliflower
½ tablespoon olive oil

¼ teaspoon kosher salt
Freshly ground black pepper

1. To make the tandoori chicken: Prick the chicken with a fork or skewer, then make three diagonal slashes in each breast, ½ inch deep and 1 inch apart. In a bowl, combine the chicken with salt, lemon juice, and turmeric. Cover and let it sit while you prepare the rest of the sauce. 2. In a bowl, mix the garlic, ginger, cardamom, cumin, paprika, and yogurt and mix thoroughly. Pour this sauce over the chicken and gently stir to coat evenly. 3. Preheat the oven to 500°F. Manage a baking sheet with parchment paper. 4. Remove the chicken from the marinade, brush it with the olive oil, and place it on the prepared baking sheet. Discard the marinade. 5. Roast it for 20-30 minutes, or until the meat reaches an internal temperature of 165°F. 6. Remove the outer green leaves and core. Roughly chop the florets. 7. In a food processor, pulse the cauliflower to resemble a crumb-like texture, almost like rice, being careful not to overpulse and make it too fine. Put the cauliflower in a bowl and set aside. 8. In a large skillet, heat the oil to shimmer, add the cauliflower and stir to coat it with the hot oil. Season with the salt and pepper. Cook for 5 minutes until the cauliflower browns and becomes tender.

Per Serving: Calories 210; Total Fat 7g; Saturated Fat 2g; Sodium 345mg; Carbs 6g; Fiber 1.5g; Sugar 3.5g; Protein 30g

Turkey Meatballs with Chickpea Pasta

Prep time: 10 minutes | Cook time: 20 minutes | Serves: 4

Cooking spray
1-pound ground turkey
1 large egg
1½ teaspoons Italian seasoning

2 teaspoons olive oil
8 ounces chickpea pasta
2 cups low-sodium tomato sauce
4 ounces Parmesan cheese (optional)

1. Boil water on high heat. 2. Preheat the broiler. Manage a baking sheet with parchment paper and spray with cooking spray. 3. In a large bowl, combine the turkey, egg, Italian seasoning, and oil. Make the meatballs and place it on the baking tray. 4. Broil until the meatballs reach an internal temperature of 165°F for 10 minutes. 5. Boil pasta, then drain. 6. In a small saucepan, heat the tomato sauce over medium-low heat and keep warm until the meatballs have finished cooking. 7. Add the cooked meatballs in the sauce and mix to coat. 8. On each plate, serve about one-quarter of the chickpea noodles. Top with tomato sauce, meatballs, and Parmesan.

Per Serving: Calories 523; Total Fat 22g; Saturated Fat 10g; Sodium 238mg; Carbs 42g; Fiber 9g; Sugar 5g; Protein 37g

Crispy Chicken Thighs with Collard Greens

Prep time: 10 minutes | Cook time: 50 minutes | Serves: 2

4 bone-in, skinless chicken thighs
1½ cups brine from Flash Pickles
½ cup whole-wheat flour
2 teaspoons paprika
1 teaspoon baking powder
3 tablespoons sesame seeds

¼ teaspoon freshly ground black pepper
Cooking spray
1 tablespoon avocado oil
½ bunch collard greens, coarsely shredded
1 garlic clove, minced

1. In a sealable bag, combine the chicken and pickle brine. Seal and marinate in refrigerate for at least 8 hours or overnight. 2. Preheat the oven to 425°F. Place a wire rack to fit over a baking sheet. 3. Using paper towels, pat dry the chicken and set aside. 4. In a bowl, add the flour with paprika, baking powder, sesame seeds, and pepper. Mix well, then toss the chicken thighs in the mixture, making sure each piece is coated. 5. Arrange the chicken pieces ½ inch apart on the wire rack over the baking sheet. Grease the chicken with cooking oil and bake for 40 to 50 minutes. 6. While the chicken rests, prepare the greens. In a skillet, heat the oil to shimmer, add the collards, toss to coat with the hot oil, for 3 minutes, or until the greens begin to wilt. Add the garlic, toss, and cook for 1 to 2 minutes.

Per Serving: Calories 562; Total Fat 34g; Saturated Fat 10g; Sodium 375mg; Carbs 23g; Fiber 6g; Sugar 0.5g; Protein 47g

Flavorful Turkey Cutlets with Zucchini

Prep time: 10 minutes | Cook time: 15 minutes | Serves: 4

¼ cup avocado oil
2 tablespoons molasses
¼ cup chopped scallions, green and white parts
1 tablespoon freshly ground black pepper
¼ teaspoon kosher salt
1 teaspoon dried thyme
½ teaspoon ground cinnamon
⅛ teaspoon ground cloves

½ teaspoon cayenne pepper
2 garlic cloves, minced
1 (1-inch) ginger, minced
¼ cup freshly squeezed lime juice
1-pound turkey breast cutlets
1 small onion, cut into ¼-inch slices
1 medium zucchini, cut into ¼-inch-by-¼-inch-by-3-inch matchsticks

1. In a large bowl, combine the oil, molasses, scallions, black pepper, salt, thyme, cinnamon, cloves, cayenne, garlic, ginger, and lime juice. Whisk until it comes together, then add the turkey cutlets, onion, and zucchini and toss to coat. 2. Preheat a cast-iron skillet or preheat the grill to medium-high. Remove the cutlets from the marinade and cook them in batches for 2 to 3 minutes per side, or until no longer pink. Transfer the cutlets to a platter and allow them to rest for 3 to 5 minutes. 3. Cook the onion and zucchini, stirring continuously, for 2 to 3 minutes, or until tender-crisp. Serve the vegetables with the turkey cutlets.

Per Serving: Calories 213; Total Fat 7.5g; Saturated Fat 2g; Sodium 167mg; Carbs 7g; Fiber 1g; Sugar 5.5g; Protein 29g

Yummy Chicken and Shrimp Jambalaya

Prep time: 30 minutes | Cook time: 2-4 hours| Serves: 6

3½-4-lb. roasting chicken, trimmed of skin nd fat, cut up
3 onions, diced
1 carrot, sliced
3-4 garlic cloves, minced
1 teaspoon dried oregano

1 teaspoon dried basil
½ teaspoon salt
⅛ teaspoon white pepper
14-oz. can crushed tomatoes
1 lb. shelled raw shrimp
2 cups cooked rice

1. Combine all ingredients instead of shrimp and rice in a slow cooker. 2. Cover. Cook on low temp setting for 2-3½ hours, or until chicken is tender. 3. Add shrimp and rice. 4. Cover. Cook on high temp setting for 15-20 minutes, or until shrimp are done.

Per Serving: Calories 354; Total Fat 7g; Saturated Fat 1.9g; Sodium 589mg; Carbs 29g; Fiber 4g; Sugar 9g; Protein 41g

Cumin Turkey Stuffed Sweet Potatoes

Prep Time: 5 minutes | Cook Time: 15 minutes |Serves: 4

4 medium sweet potatoes
2 tablespoons extra-virgin olive oil
1 pound 93% lean ground turkey
2 teaspoons ground cumin

1 teaspoon chili powder
½ teaspoon salt
½ teaspoon freshly ground black pepper

1. Fork-prick the potatoes, then microwave them for 10 minutes on high power or on the potato setting. 2. Over medium heat, preheat a medium skillet. When the skillet is heated, add the oil, turkey, cumin, chili powder, salt, and pepper. Stir and break up the meat as necessary. 3. The potatoes should be taken out of the microwave and cut in half lengthwise. With a spoon, push the centers of each half, then evenly distribute cooked turkey within.

Per Serving: Calories 318; Total Fat 13g; Saturated Fat 3g; Sodium 443mg; Carbs 27g; Fiber 4g; Sugar 8g; Protein 23g

Cheese Turkey Zucchini Spaghetti

Prep Time: 5 minutes | Cook Time: 20 minutes |Serves: 4

1 (10-ounce) package zucchini noodles
2 tablespoons extra-virgin olive oil, divided
1 pound 93% lean ground turkey

½ teaspoon dried oregano
2 cups low-sodium spaghetti sauce
½ cup shredded sharp Cheddar cheese

1. Dry off the zucchini noodles with two paper towels. 2. 1 tablespoon of olive oil should be heated over medium heat in a medium oven-safe pan. Add the zucchini noodles after they're heated. 3 minutes, stirring once halfway through cooking. 3. Ground turkey, oregano, and the last tablespoon of oil are added. Cook for 7 to 10 minutes, breaking up any clumps and stirring as necessary. 4. Stir in the spaghetti sauce after adding it to the pan. 5. Place the oven rack in the middle if your oven's broiler is on the top shelf. Broiler: Turn on high. 6. Then add cheese, broil for 5 minutes, or until the cheese is bubbling, on top of the mixture.

Per Serving: Calories 356; Total Fat 14g; Saturated Fat 3g; Sodium 291mg; Carbs 30g; Fiber 2g; Sugar 7g; Protein 26g

Tasty Chicken with Tomato & Olives

Prep Time: 5 minutes | Cook Time: 35 minutes |Serves: 4

2 tablespoons olive oil
1 cup chopped onion
1 teaspoon minced garlic
1½ cups chopped green peppers
1 pound boneless, skinless chicken breast,

cut into 4 pieces
2 cups diced tomatoes
1 teaspoon oregano
½ cup pitted, chopped kalamata olives

1. In a big skillet, warm the olive oil over medium heat. Sauté the peppers, onions, and garlic for approximately 5 minutes, or until the onions are transparent. 2. Add the chicken bits. Cook until light brown on each side for about 5 minutes. 3. Add the oregano and tomatoes. Simmer for 20 minutes on low heat. 4. Before serving, add the olives and simmer for an additional 10 minutes.

Per Serving: Calories 310; Total Fat 15g; Saturated Fat 3g; Sodium 433mg; Carbs 32g; Fiber 4g; Sugar 10g; Protein 12g

Lime-Coconut Chicken and Asparagus

Prep Time: 5 minutes | Cook Time: 15 minutes |Serves: 4

1 tablespoon coconut oil
4 (4-ounce) boneless, skinless chicken breasts
½ teaspoon salt
1 red bell pepper, cut into ¼-inch-thick slices
16 asparagus spears, bottom ends trimmed

1 cup unsweetened coconut milk
2 tablespoons freshly squeezed lime juice
½ teaspoon garlic powder
¼ teaspoon red pepper flakes
¼ cup chopped fresh cilantro

1. Over medium-low heat, warm the oil in a large skillet. Add the chicken once it is heated. 2. Add salt to the chicken to season it. Flip after 5 minutes of cooking. 3. Add the bell pepper and asparagus to the pan after pushing the chicken to one side. Cook for 5 minutes with the lid on. 4. In the meantime, combine the coconut milk, garlic powder, lime juice, and red pepper flakes in a small bowl. 5. The coconut milk mixture should be added to the skillet and boiled for two to three minutes on high heat. 6. Top with the cilantro.

Per Serving: Calories 276; Total Fat 12g; Saturated Fat 5g; Sodium 622mg; Carbs 30g; Fiber 2g; Sugar 10g; Protein 13g

Chicken with Balsamic Onion Sauce

Prep Time: 5 minutes | Cook Time: 30 minutes |Serves: 4

1 pound boneless, skinless chicken breasts, cut into
4 pieces Pinch salt
¼ teaspoon pepper
1 tablespoon butter
1 tablespoon olive oil

¼ cup red onion, chopped
2 teaspoons finely chopped garlic
3 tablespoons balsamic vinegar
1½ cups low-sodium chicken broth
1 teaspoon oregano

1. Salt and pepper the chicken as desired. 2. In a big skillet, melt butter and olive oil over medium heat. Add the chicken and cook for approximately 5 minutes on each side, or until browned. 3. Cook for 12 minutes on low heat. Place on a dish, cover, and maintain warm. 4. Garlic and red onions should be added to the skillet. For three minutes, sauté over medium heat while scraping away the browned parts. 5. Bring to a boil after including the balsamic vinegar. Stirring continuously, bring to a boil for 3 minutes or until reduced to a glaze. 6. Including the chicken broth Boil until the liquid is reduced to approximately 3/4 cup. Add the chopped oregano after removing the sauce from the heat. Serve the chicken with sauce right away.

Per Serving: Calories 283; Total Fat 13g; Saturated Fat 4g; Sodium 356mg; Carbs 28g; Fiber 2g; Sugar 8g; Protein 12g

Wine-Braised Chicken with Spaghetti

Prep Time: 5 minutes | Cook Time: 25 minutes | Serves: 4

2 teaspoons olive oil
½ cup chopped onion
2 cloves garlic, minced
4 chicken thighs, skin removed
½ cup dry red wine
1 (14½-ounce) can unsalted diced tomatoes, undrained
1 teaspoon dried parsley

½ teaspoon dried oregano
¼ teaspoon pepper
⅛ teaspoon sugar
¼ cup grated Parmesan cheese
4 cups cooked spaghetti
2 teaspoons extra-virgin olive oil

1. Add two teaspoons of olive oil to a deep, nonstick pan that is already hot over medium-high heat. Add the onion and cook for 2 to 3 minutes, or until translucent. 2. Chicken thighs should be sautéed for 3 minutes on each side, or until just barely browned, after adding the garlic. Take the thighs out of the pan. 3. Wine, tomatoes, their juices, parsley, oregano, pepper, and sugar should all be added to the pan. Stir well then bring to a boil. 4. Return the chicken to the pan. On top, grate some Parmesan cheese. For 10 minutes, simmer with a cover on and reduced heat. 5. For an additional 10 minutes, remove the cover. 6. Put 1 cup of the cooked pasta on each of the 4 dishes before serving. Add a chicken thigh on the top of each serving. Divide sauce between dishes. Drizzle ½ teaspoon extra-virgin olive oil over top of each dish and serve.

Per Serving: Calories 770; Total Fat 38g; Saturated Fat 10g; Sodium 367mg; Carbs 63g; Fiber 11g; Sugar 16g; Protein 46g

Chicken and Zucchini Stuffed Spaghetti Squash

Prep Time: 5 minutes | Cook Time: 40 minutes | Serves: 4

1 (3-pound) spaghetti squash, halved lengthwise and seeded
1½ teaspoons ground cumin, divided
Avocado oil cooking spray

4 (4-ounce) boneless, skinless chicken breasts
1 large zucchini, diced
¾ cup canned red enchilada sauce
¾ cup shredded Cheddar or mozzarella cheese

1. Preheat the oven to 400°F. 2. Put the squash cut-side down on a baking pan after seasoning with ½ tsp cumin. Bake for 25 to 30 minutes. 3. In the meantime, preheat a large skillet over low heat. Spray the heated cooking surface with cooking spray before adding the zucchini, chicken breasts, and 1 teaspoon of cumin. Per side, cook the chicken for 4 to 5 minutes. When you turn the chicken, stir the zucchini. 4. Zucchini should be added to a medium bowl and left aside. When the chicken is cool enough to handle, remove it from the skillet and let it rest for 10 minutes. The chicken should be diced or shredded. 5. Add the enchilada sauce to the big bowl with the chicken and zucchini. 6. After removing the squash from the oven, turn it over, and create thin strands out of it with a fork. 7. Scoop the chicken mixture over the squash halves, then sprinkle cheese over top. When the cheese is bubbling, put the squash back in the oven and broil for an additional 2 to 5 minutes.

Per Serving: Calories 436; Total Fat 12g; Saturated Fat 4g; Sodium 503mg; Carbs 66g; Fiber 8g; Sugar 7g; Protein 18g

White Wine Braised Chicken with Mushroom & Asparagus

Prep Time: 5 minutes | Cook Time: 15 minutes |Serves: 4

4 boneless, skinless chicken breast halves
½ tablespoon butter
1 tablespoon olive oil
1 teaspoon garlic, finely chopped
½ cup onion, finely chopped
10 ounces' asparagus spears, cut diagonally in 2" pieces

½ pound mushrooms
¼ cup dry white wine
¼ cup water
1 tablespoon chopped parsley
Salt and pepper, to taste

1. The chicken should be pounded to a thickness of 1". 2. Over medium heat, combine butter and olive oil to melt. Add the minced garlic and onion, and cook for one to two minutes. 3. Chicken should be added and cooked for 5 minutes, or until both sides are browned. Remove and reserve the chicken. 4. Add the mushrooms and asparagus to the skillet. 2 to 3 minutes of cooking. 5. Add chicken in the pan with water and white wine. swiftly bring to a boil. To decrease the liquid, boil it for two minutes. 6. Warm up less. The chicken and veggies should be tender after three minutes of simmering with the lid on. Serve with freshly chopped parsley, salt, and pepper to taste.
Per Serving: Calories 406; Total Fat 10g; Saturated Fat 3g; Sodium 237mg; Carbs 48g; Fiber 8g; Sugar 4g; Protein 37g

Cheesy Rice & Chicken Stuffed Bell Peppers

Prep Time: 5 minutes | Cook Time: 30 minutes |Serves: 4

2 large red bell peppers
2 teaspoons extra-virgin olive oil, divided
½ cup uncooked brown rice or quinoa
4 (4-ounce) boneless, skinless chicken breasts
¼ teaspoon garlic powder

¼ teaspoon onion powder
⅛ teaspoon dried thyme
½ teaspoon dried oregano
½ cup crumbled feta

1. Cut the bell peppers in half and remove the seeds. 2. 1 teaspoon of olive oil should be warmed up in a large skillet over low heat. When the skillet is heated, add the bell pepper halves, cut-side up. Cook for 20 minutes with a cover on. 3. The rice should be prepared as directed on the packaging. 4. Cut the chicken into 1-inch pieces while you wait. 4. The remaining 1 teaspoon of olive oil should be heated over low heat in a medium pan. Add the chicken once it is heated. 5. Garlic powder, onion powder, thyme, and oregano are used to season the chicken. 6. Cook thoroughly for 5 minutes, stirring periodically. 7. Combine the cooked rice and chicken in a large bowl. Fill each pepper half with a quarter of the chicken and rice mixture, cover, and simmer for 10 minutes at a low heat. 8. Add 2 tablespoons of feta crumbles to the top of each pepper half.
Per Serving: Calories 382; Total Fat 12g; Saturated Fat 5g; Sodium 594mg; Carbs 52g; Fiber 3.2g; Sugar 8g; Protein 16g

Teriyaki Chicken with Broccoli & Cauliflower Rice

Prep Time: 5 minutes | Cook Time: 20 minutes | Serves: 4

For the Sauce:
½ cup water
2 tablespoons low-sodium soy sauce
2 tablespoons honey
1 tablespoon rice vinegar
¼ teaspoon garlic powder
Pinch ground ginger

1 tablespoon cornstarch
For the Entrée:
1 tablespoon sesame oil
4 (4-ounce) boneless, skinless chicken breasts, cut into bite-size cubes
1 (12-ounce) bag frozen broccoli
1 (12-ounce) bag frozen cauliflower rice

To make the sauce: 1. Water, soy sauce, honey, garlic powder, rice vinegar, and ginger should all be combined in a small saucepan. Cornstarch should be added and whisked in completely. 2. Bring the teriyaki sauce to a boil over medium heat. To thicken, let the sauce simmer for one minute. The sauce should be turned off the heat and kept aside.

To make the entrée: 1. A big skillet should be heated on low heat. Add the oil and the chicken once it is heated. Stirring occasionally, cook the chicken for 5 to 7 minutes, or until it is well done. 2. As directed on the packaging, steam the broccoli and cauliflower rice in the microwave. 3. Four equal pieces of cauliflower rice should be made. Each portion should include a quarter of the chicken, broccoli, and teriyaki sauce on top.

Per Serving: Calories 339; Total Fat 11g; Saturated Fat 2g; Sodium 209mg; Carbs 47g; Fiber 4g; Sugar 20g; Protein 14g

Chapter 5 Meat Recipes

Big Beef Stew

Prep time: 25 minutes | Cook time: 9 hours | Serves: 8

3 lb. beef roast, cubed, trimmed of fat
1 large onion, sliced
1 teaspoon dried parsley flakes
1 medium green pepper, sliced
3 ribs celery, sliced

4 medium carrots, sliced
28-oz. can tomatoes with juice, undrained
1 garlic clove, minced
2 cups water

1. Combine all ingredients. 2. Cover. Cook on high 1 hour. Reduce heat to low and cook 8 hours. 3. Serve on rice or noodles.

Per Serving: Calories 224; Total Fat 7g; Saturated Fat 2.1g; Sodium 248mg; Carbs 12g; Fiber 3g; Sugar 7g; Protein 28g

Delicious Round Steak and Celery

Prep time: 25 minutes | Cook time: 8 hours | Serves: 6

1 small onion, sliced
1 rib celery, chopped
1 medium green bell pepper, sliced in rings
2 lbs. round steak, trimmed of fat
2 tablespoon chopped fresh parsley
1 tablespoon Worcestershire sauce

1 tablespoon dry mustard
1 tablespoon chili powder
2 cups canned tomatoes
2 teaspoon dry minced garlic
½ teaspoon salt
¼ teaspoon pepper

1. Put half of onion, green pepper, and celery in a slow cooker. 2. Cut steak into serving-size pieces. Place steak pieces in slow cooker. 3. Put remaining onion, green pepper, and celery over steak. 4. Combine remaining ingredients. Pour over meat. 5. Cover. Cook on low 8 hours. 6. Serve over noodles or rice.

Per Serving: Calories 222; Total Fat 7g; Saturated Fat 2.3g; Sodium 414mg; Carbs 8g; Fiber 2g; Sugar 5g; Protein 30g

Soy Beef Steak Stew

Prep time: 25 minutes | Cook time: 6-7 hours | Serves: 8

1½-2 lbs. beef round steak, cut in 3" × 1" strips, trimmed of fat
2 Tablespoon canola oil
¼ cup soy sauce
1 garlic clove, minced
1 cup chopped onion
1 teaspoon sugar

¼ teaspoon pepper
¼ teaspoon ground ginger
2 large green peppers, cut in strips
4 medium tomatoes cut in eighths, or 16 oz. can diced tomatoes
½ cup cold water
1 Tablespoon cornstarch

1. Brown beef in oil in saucepan. Transfer to slow cooker. 2. Combine soy sauce, garlic, onions, sugar, salt, pepper, and ginger. Pour over meat. 3. Cover. Cook on low for temp setting for 5-6 hours. 4. Add in tomatoes and peppers. Cook 1 hour longer. 5. Mix water and cornstarch slurry. Stir into slow cooker pot. Cook on high temp setting until thickened, about 10 minutes. 6. Serve over rice or noodles.

Per Serving: Calories 174; Total Fat 8g; Saturated Fat 1.5g; Sodium 546mg; Carbs 10g; Fiber 2g; Sugar 6g; Protein 17g

Spicy Steak and Mushroom

Prep time: 20 minutes | Cook time: 6-8 hours| Serves: 6

1 lb. round steak, sliced thin, trimmed of fat
3 Tablespoon light soy sauce
½ teaspoon ground ginger
1 garlic clove, minced
1 medium green pepper, thinly sliced

4-oz. can mushroom, drained, or 1 cup sliced fresh mushrooms
1 medium onion, thinly sliced
½ teaspoon crushed red pepper

1. Add all ingredients in a slow cooker pot. 2. Cover. Cook on low 6-8 hours. 3. Serve as steak sandwiches topped with provolone cheese, or over rice.

Per Serving: Calories 122; Total Fat 4g; Saturated Fat 1.2g; Sodium 368mg; Carbs 6g; Fiber 2g; Sugar 3g; Protein 16g

Mexican-Style Chuck Roast

Prep time: 20 minutes | Cook time: 8-10 hours| Serves: 6

3 lb. boneless chuck roast, trimmed of fat
1 garlic clove, minced
1 Tablespoon canola oil
2-3 medium onions, sliced

2-3 sweet green and red peppers, sliced
16-oz. jar salsa
2 14½-oz. cans Mexican-style stewed tomatoes

1. Brown roast and garlic in oil in skillet. Place in slow cooker. 2. Add onions and peppers. 3. Mix salsa and tomatoes and pour over in slow cooker. 4. Cover. Cook on low 8-10 hours.5. Slice meat to serve.

Per Serving: Calories 327; Total Fat 11g; Saturated Fat 3.1g; Sodium 565mg; Carbs 19g; Fiber 5g; Sugar 12g; Protein 38g

Beef, Potato and Vegetables Stew

Prep time: 30 minutes | Cook time: 6-8 hours| Serves: 8

1½ lbs. beef stewing meat, cubed, trimmed of fat
2 10-oz. pkg. frozen vegetables—carrots, corn, peas
4 large potatoes, unpeeled, cubed
1 bay leaf
1 medium onion, chopped
15-oz. can stewed tomatoes of your choice—Italian,

Mexican, or regular
8-oz. can tomato sauce
2 Tablespoon Worcestershire sauce
1 teaspoon salt
¼ teaspoon pepper

1. Put meat on bottom of slow cooker. Layer frozen vegetables and potatoes over meat. 2. Mix all remaining ingredients and pour over other ingredients. 3. Cover. Cook on low 6-8 hours.

Per Serving: Calories 259; Total Fat 3g; Saturated Fat 1g; Sodium 506mg; Carbs 39g; Fiber 6g; Sugar 9g; Protein 19g

Beef Tapioca Stew

Prep time: 25 minutes | Cook time: 4-10 hours| Serves: 5

1-2 lbs. beef roast, cubed, trimmed of fat
1 teaspoon salt
¼ teaspoon pepper
2 cups water
2 small carrots, sliced

2 small onions, sliced
4-6 small potatoes, unpeeled, chunked
¼ cup quick-cooking tapioca
1 bay leaf
10-oz. pkg. frozen peas, or mixed vegetables

1. Brown beef in saucepan. Place in slow cooker. 2. Sprinkle with salt and pepper. Add remaining ingredients except frozen vegetables. Mix well. 3. Cover. Cook on low temp setting for temp setting for8-10 hours, or on high 4-5 hours. Add vegetables during last 1-2 hours of cooking.
Per Serving: Calories 257; Total Fat 4g; Saturated Fat 1.1g; Sodium 567mg; Carbs 36g; Fiber 6g; Sugar 7g; Protein 20g

Beef Carrot Stew

Prep time: 20 minutes | Cook time: 7-8 hours| Serves: 6

1½ lbs. stewing meat, cubed, trimmed of fat
2¼ cups no-added-salt tomato juice
10½-oz. can low-sodium beef broth
1 cup chopped celery
2 cups sliced carrots

4 tablespoon quick-cooking tapioca
1 medium onion, chopped
¼ teaspoon salt
¼ teaspoon pepper

1. Add all ingredients in a slow cooker pot. 2. Cover. Cook on low 7-8 hours.
Per Serving: Calories 193; Total Fat 4g; Saturated Fat 1.4g; Sodium 519mg; Carbs 17g; Fiber 3g; Sugar 7g; Protein 21g

Meat and Tomato Stew

Prep time: 15 minutes | Cook time: 6-10 hours| Serves: 6

2 lbs. stewing meat, cubed, trimmed of fat
1 envelope sodium-free dry onion soup mix
29-oz. can peeled, or crushed, tomatoes
1 teaspoon dried oregano

garlic powder to taste
2 Tablespoon canola oil
2 Tablespoon wine vinegar

1. Layer meat evenly in bottom of slow cooker. 2. Combine soup mix, tomatoes, spices, oil, and vinegar in bowl. Blend with spoon. Pour over meat. 3. Cover. Cook on high temp setting for 6 hours, or low 8-10 hours.
Per Serving: Calories 237; Total Fat 10g; Saturated Fat 2.1g; Sodium 252mg; Carbs 10g; Fiber 2g; Sugar 5g; Protein 25g

Spicy Beef Stew

Prep time: 25 minutes | Cook time: 4-6 hours| Serves: 6

2 lbs. sirloin, or stewing meat, cubed, trimmed of fat
2 Tablespoon canola oil
1 large onion, diced
2 garlic cloves, minced
1½ cups water
1 Tablespoon dried parsley flakes
1 beef bouillon cube

1 teaspoon ground cumin
¼ teaspoon salt
3 medium carrots, sliced
1 lb. frozen green beans
1 lb. frozen corn
4-oz. can diced green chilies

1. Sear meat, onion, and garlic in oil in a pan until meat is brown no longer pink. 2.Place all ingredients in slow cooker pot. 3. Cover. Cook on high temp setting for 30 minutes. Lower the heat and cook 4-6 hours.
Per Serving: Calories 322; Total Fat 11g; Saturated Fat 2.2g; Sodium 554mg; Carbs 30g; Fiber 7g; Sugar 10g; Protein 28g

Round Steak and Wild Rice Casserole

Prep time: 35 minutes | Cook time: 6-8 hours| Serves: 8

1 cup wild rice, rinsed and drained
1 cup celery, chopped
1 cup carrots, chopped
2 4-oz. cans mushrooms, stems and pieces, drained
1 large onion, chopped
1 clove garlic, minced

½ cup slivered almonds
1 beef bouillon cube
1¼ teaspoon seasoned salt
2 lbs. boneless round steak, cut into 1-inch cubes, trimmed of fat
3 cups water

1. Place ingredients in order listed in slow cooker. 2. Cover. Cook on low temp setting for 6-8 hours or until rice is tender. Stir before serving.
Per Serving: Calories 264; Total Fat 9g; Saturated Fat 1.7g; Sodium 615mg; Carbs 23g; Fiber 4g; Sugar 4g; Protein 24g

Beef Peas Stew

Prep time: 30 minutes | Cook time: 8 hours| Serves: 6

2 lb. beef roast, cubed, trimmed of fat
2 cups sliced carrots
2 cups diced potatoes, unpeeled
1 medium onion, sliced
1½ cups frozen or fresh peas
2 teaspoon quick-cooking tapioca

½ teaspoon salt
½ teaspoon pepper
8-oz. can tomato sauce
1 cup water
1 Tablespoon brown sugar

1. Combine beef and vegetables in the slow cooker. Sprinkle with tapioca, salt, and pepper. 2. Combine tomato sauce and water. Pour over ingredients in slow cooker. Sprinkle with brown sugar. 3. Cover. Cook on low 8 hours.
Per Serving: Calories 271; Total Fat 6g; Saturated Fat 1.9g; Sodium 539mg; Carbs 26g; Fiber 5g; Sugar 11g; Protein 28g

Beef and Lima Beans Stew

Prep time: 30 minutes | Cook time: 8 hours | Serves: 8

2 lbs. stewing beef, cubed, trimmed of fat
2 cups diced carrots
2 cups diced potatoes, unpeeled
2 medium onions, chopped
1 cup chopped celery
10-oz. pkg. lima beans

2 teaspoon quick-cooking tapioca
1 teaspoon salt
½ teaspoon pepper
8-oz. can tomato sauce
1 cup water
1 tablespoon brown sugar

1. Place beef in bottom of slow cooker. Add vegetables. 2. Sprinkle tapioca, salt, and pepper over ingredients. 3. Mix together tomato sauce and water. Pour over top. 4. Sprinkle brown sugar over all. 5. Cover. Cook on low 8 hours.
Per Serving: Calories 229; Total Fat 5g; Saturated Fat 1.4g; Sodium 558mg; Carbs 25g; Fiber 5g; Sugar 8g; Protein 22g

Traditional Beef Pot Roast

Prep time: 30 minutes | Cook time: 10-12 hours | Serves: 10

2 medium potatoes, cubed, or 2 medium sweet potatoes, cubed
8 small carrots, cut in small chunks
2 small onions, cut in wedges
2 ribs celery, chopped
2½-3 lb. beef chuck, or pot roast, trimmed of fat

2 tablespoons canola oil
¾ cup water, dry wine, or tomato juice
1 tablespoon Worcestershire sauce
1 teaspoon instant beef bouillon granules
1 teaspoon dried basil

1. Place vegetables in bottom of slow cooker. 2. Brown roast in oil in skillet. Place on top of vegetables. 3. Combine water, Worcestershire sauce, bouillon, and basil. Pour over meat and vegetables. 4. Cover. Cook on low 10-12 hours.
Per Serving: Calories 233; Total Fat 9g; Saturated Fat 2.1g; Sodium 231mg; Carbs 16g; Fiber 3g; Sugar 5g; Protein 22g

Easy Chuck Roast and Veggies Stew

Prep time: 20 minutes | Cook time: 6-8 hours | Serves: 6

3-4 lb. chuck roast, trimmed of fat
4 medium potatoes, cubed, unpeeled
4 medium carrots, sliced, or 1 lb. baby carrots

2 celery ribs, sliced thin
1 envelope dry onion soup mix
3 cups water

1. Put roast, potatoes, carrots, and celery in slow cooker. 2. Add onion soup mix and water. 3. Cover. Cook on low 6-8 hours.
Per Serving: Calories 325; Total Fat 8g; Saturated Fat 2.9g; Sodium 560mg; Carbs 26g; Fiber 4g; Sugar 6g; Protein 35g

Simple Pot Roast

Prep time: 10 minutes | Cook time: 10-12 hours | Serves: 8

3 potatoes, thinly sliced
2 large carrots, thinly sliced
1 onion, thinly sliced
1 teaspoon salt

½ teaspoon pepper
3-4 lb. pot roast, trimmed of fat
½ cup water

1. Put vegetables in the slow cooker. Stir in salt and pepper. Add roast. Pour in water. 2. Cover. Cook on low 10-12 hours.

Per Serving: Calories 219; Total Fat 6g; Saturated Fat 2.2g; Sodium 361mg; Carbs 14g; Fiber 2g; Sugar 3g; Protein 26g

Beef, Turnip and Green Beans Stew

Prep time: 35 minutes | Cook time: 6-8 hours | Serves: 6

1 lb. stewing beef
1 cup cubed turnip
2 medium potatoes, cubed, unpeeled
1 large onion, sliced
1 garlic clove, minced
2 large carrots, sliced
½ cup green beans, cut up
½ cup peas

1 bay leaf
½ teaspoon dried thyme
1 teaspoon chopped parsley
2 Tablespoon tomato paste
2 Tablespoon celery leaves
¼ teaspoon salt
¼ teaspoon pepper
1 qt., or 2 14½-oz. cans, lower-sodium beef broth

1. Place meat, vegetables, and seasonings in the slow cooker. Pour broth over all. 2. Cover. Cook on low 6-8 hours.

Per Serving: Calories 175; Total Fat 3g; Saturated Fat 0.9g; Sodium 466mg; Carbs 21g; Fiber 5g; Sugar 6g; Protein 16g

Slow Cooked Veal and Green Peppers

Prep time: 15 minutes | Cook time: 4-7 hours | Serves: 4

1½ lbs. boneless veal, cubed
3 green bell peppers, quartered
2 onions, thinly sliced
½ lb. fresh mushrooms, sliced

1 teaspoon salt
½ teaspoon dried basil
2 cloves garlic, minced
28-oz. can tomatoes

1. Add all ingredients in a slow cooker pot. 2. Cover. Cook on low 7 hours, or on high 4 hours. 3. Serve over rice or noodles.

Per Serving: Calories 194; Total Fat 3g; Saturated Fat 0.9g; Sodium 555mg; Carbs 16g; Fiber 4g; Sugar 9g; Protein 26g

Homemade Pot Roast and Vegetables Stew

Prep time: 30 minutes | Cook time: 4-10 hours | Serves: 6

3-4 lb. bottom round, rump, or arm roast, trimmed of fat
¼ teaspoon salt
2-3 teaspoon pepper
2 Tablespoon flour
¼ cup cold water
1 teaspoon Kitchen Bouquet, or gravy

browning seasoning sauce
1 garlic clove, minced
2 medium onions, cut in wedges
4 medium potatoes, cubed, unpeeled
2 carrots, quartered
1 green bell pepper, sliced

1. Place roast in slow cooker. Sprinkle with salt and pepper. 2. Make paste of flour and cold water. Stir in Kitchen Bouquet and spread over roast. 3. Add garlic, onions, potatoes, carrots, and green pepper. 4. Cover. Cook on low temp setting for 8-10 hours, or high 4-5 hours. 5. Taste and adjust seasonings before serving.
Per Serving: Calories 336; Total Fat 8g; Saturated Fat 2.9g; Sodium 577mg; Carbs 28g; Fiber 4g; Sugar 7g; Protein 36g

Classic "Smothered" Steak

Prep time: 20 minutes | Cook time: 8 hours | Serves: 6

1½-lb. chuck, or round, steak, cut into strips, trimmed of fat
⅓ cup flour
¼ teaspoon pepper
1 large onion, sliced

1 green pepper, sliced
14½-oz. can of stewed tomatoes
4-oz. can of mushrooms, drained
2 Tablespoon soy sauce
10-oz. pkg. frozen French-style green beans

1. Layer steak in bottom of slow cooker. Sprinkle with flour, salt, and pepper. Stir well to coat steak. 2. Add remaining ingredients. Mix together gently. 3. Cover. Cook on low 8 hours. 4. Serve over rice.
Per Serving: Calories 222; Total Fat 6g; Saturated Fat 1.7g; Sodium 613mg; Carbs 19g; Fiber 4g; Sugar 7g; Protein 25g

Chili Beef and Beans Stew

Prep time: 20 minutes | Cook time: 6-9 hours | Serves: 8

1 tablespoon prepared mustard
1 tablespoon chili powder
½ teaspoon salt
¼ teaspoon pepper
1½-lb. boneless round steak, cut into thin slices,

trimmed of fat
2 14½-oz. cans diced tomatoes, undrained
1 medium onion, chopped
1 beef bouillon cube, crushed
16-oz. can kidney beans, rinsed and drained

1. Combine mustard, chili powder, salt, and pepper. Add beef slices and toss to coat. Place meat in slow cooker. 2. Add tomatoes, onion, and bouillon. 3. Cover. Cook on low 6-8 hours. 4. Stir in beans. Cook 30 minutes longer. 5. Serve over rice.
Per Serving: Calories 182; Total Fat 4g; Saturated Fat 1.3g; Sodium 582mg; Carbs 16g; Fiber 4g; Sugar 6g; Protein 21g

Three Beans Burrito Bake

Prep time: 20 minutes | Cook time: 8-10 hours | Serves: 8

1 tablespoon canola oil
1 onion, chopped
1 green bell pepper, chopped
2 garlic cloves, minced
16-oz. can pinto beans, drained
16-oz. can kidney beans, drained
15-oz. can black beans, drained
4-oz. can sliced black olives, drained

4-oz. can green chilies
2 15-oz. cans no-added-salt diced tomatoes
1 teaspoon chili powder
1 teaspoon ground cumin
6 6" flour tortillas
1 cup shredded Co-Jack cheese
sour cream

1. Sauté onions, peppers, and garlic in skillet in oil. 2. Add beans and olives, chilies, tomatoes, chili powder, and cumin. 3. In greased slow cooker pot, layer ¾ cup vegetables, a tortilla, ⅓ cheese. Repeat layers ending with sauce. 4. Cover. Cook on low 8-10 hours. 5. Serve with sour cream.

Per Serving: Calories 346; Total Fat 11g; Saturated Fat 3.3g; Sodium 573mg; Carbs 48g; Fiber 12g; Sugar 8g; Protein 16g

Authentic Beef Stew

Prep time: 25 minutes | Cook time: 10-12 hours | Serves: 6

2 lbs. stewing beef, cut in 1-inch cubes, trimmed of fat
2 tablespoon canola oil
10¾-oz. can of condensed golden cream of mushroom soup
1 teaspoon Worcestershire sauce
⅓ cup dry red wine
½ teaspoon dried oregano

¼ teaspoon salt
½ teaspoon pepper
½ cup chopped onions
½ cup chopped carrots
4-oz. can mushroom pieces, drained
½ cup cold water
¼ cup flour

1. Brown meat in oil in saucepan. Transfer to slow cooker. 2. Mix together soup, Worcestershire sauce, wine, oregano, salt and pepper, onions, carrots, and mushrooms. Pour over meat. 3. Cover. Cook on low 10-12 hours. 4. Combine water and flour. Stir into beef mixture. Turn cooker to high. 5. Cook until thickened and bubbly. 6. Serve over noodles.

Per Serving: Calories 266; Total Fat 12g; Saturated Fat 2.5g; Sodium 585mg; Carbs 12g; Fiber 2g; Sugar 2g; Protein 26g

Juicy Steak and Mushroom

Prep time: 20 minutes | Cook time: 9-10 hours | Serves: 4

1½-lb. round steak, cut ½-¾-inch thick, trimmed of fat
¼ cup flour
½ teaspoon salt
¼ teaspoon pepper
¼ teaspoon paprika
2 medium onions, sliced

4-oz. can of sliced mushrooms, drained
½ cup beef broth
2 teaspoon Worcestershire sauce
2 tablespoon flour
3 tablespoon water

1. Mix together ¼ cup flour, salt, pepper, and paprika. 2. Cut steak into 5-6 pieces. Dredge steak in seasoned flour until lightly coated. 3. Layer half of onions, half of the steak, and half of mushrooms into cooker. Repeat. 4. Combine beef broth and Worcestershire sauce. Pour over mixture in slow cooker. 5. Cover. Cook on low 8-10 hours. 6. Place steak to serving platter and keep warm. Mix together 2 tablespoons of flour with water. Stir into drippings and cook on high temp setting until thickened, about 10 minutes. Pour over steak and serve.
Per Serving: Calories 295; Total Fat 8g; Saturated Fat 2.6g; Sodium 601mg; Carbs 18g; Fiber 3g; Sugar 6g; Protein 36g

Traditional Stroganoff Steak

Prep time: 15 minutes | Cook time: 3-7 hours | Serves: 6

2 tablespoon flour
½ teaspoon garlic powder
½ teaspoon pepper
¼ teaspoon paprika
1¾-lb. boneless beef round steak, trimmed of fat
10¾-oz. can reduced-sodium, 98% fat-free cream of

mushroom soup
½ cup water
1 envelope sodium-free dried onion soup mix
9-oz. jar sliced mushrooms, drained
½ cup fat-free sour cream
1 tablespoon minced fresh parsley

1. Add flour, garlic powder, pepper, and paprika in a slow cooker. 2. Cut meat into 1½ × ½-inch strips. Stir in flour mix and toss until meat is well coated. 3. Add mushroom soup, water, and soup mix. Stir until well blended. 4. Cover. Cook on high 3-3½ hours, or low 6-7 hours. 5. Stir in mushrooms, sour cream, and parsley. Cover and cook on high temp setting for 10-15 minutes, or until heated through.
Per Serving: Calories 256; Total Fat 7g; Saturated Fat 2.4g; Sodium 390mg; Carbs 17g; Fiber 2g; Sugar 5g; Protein 29g

Beef, Beans and Corn Stew

Prep Time: 25 minutes | Cook Time: 4-6½ hours |Serves: 6

2 lbs. sirloin, or stewing meat, cubed, trimmed of fat
2 tbsps. canola oil
1 large onion, diced
2 garlic cloves, minced
1½ cups water
1 tbsp. dried parsley flakes
1 beef bouillon cube

1 tsp. ground cumin
¼ tsp. salt
3 medium carrots, sliced
1 lb. frozen green beans
1 lb. frozen corn
4-oz. can diced green chilies

1. Oil in a pot should be used to brown the beef, onion, and garlic until the meat is no longer pink. Add to a slow cooker. 2. Add additional ingredients and stir. 3. Cover. Cook for 30 minutes on high. Cook for four to six hours on low heat.

Per Serving: Calories 390; Total Fat 12g; Saturated Fat 2g; Sodium 769mg; Carbs 35g; Fiber 10g; Sugar 5g; Protein 37g

Beef and Cabbage Stew

Prep time: 40 minutes | Cook time: 8-10 hours | Serves: 8

2 medium carrots, sliced
1 medium onion, sliced
2 cups water
1 tablespoon vinegar
1 celery rib, sliced
3 lb. boneless chuck roast, trimmed of fat
¼ teaspoon pepper
1 dry onion soup mix

1 bay leaf
Half head of cabbage, cut in wedges
2 tablespoons melted margarine, or butter
2 tablespoons flour
1 tablespoon dried minced onion
2 tablespoons prepared horseradish
½ teaspoon salt

1. Place carrots, onion, and celery in slow cooker. Place roast on top. Sprinkle with pepper. Add soup mix with water, vinegar, and bay leaf. 2. Cover. Cook on low temp setting for 7-9 hours. 3. Discard bay leaf. Add cabbage to juice in slow cooker. 4. Cover. Cook on high temp setting for 1 hour, or until cabbage is tender. 5. Melt margarine in saucepan. Stir in flour and onion. 6. Add 1½ cups liquid from slow cooker. Stir in horseradish and ½ teaspoon salt. Bring to boil. 7. Cook over low setting until thicken and smooth, about 2 minutes. Return to cooker and blend with remaining sauce in cooker. 8. When blended, serve over or alongside meat and vegetables.

Per Serving: Calories 234; Total Fat 9g; Saturated Fat 2.7g; Sodium 607mg; Carbs 11g; Fiber 3g; Sugar 6g; Protein 26g

Flank Steak with Peppers Stew

Prep Time: 15 minutes | Cook Time: 5-8 hours | Serves: 10

3 bell peppers—one red, one orange, and one yellow pepper (or any combination of colors), cut into ¼"-thick slices
2 garlic cloves, sliced
1 large onion, sliced
1 tsp. ground cumin
½ tsp. dried oregano

1 bay leaf
3-lb. beef flank steak, cut in ¼-½"-thick slices across the grain
Salt to taste
14½-oz. can diced tomatoes in juice
Jalapeño chilies, sliced, optional

1. In a slow cooker, combine sliced peppers, garlic, onion, cumin, oregano, and bay leaf. To blend, gently stir. 2. Place pieces of steak over the veggie mixture. Use salt to season. 3. Top with tomatoes and their juice. If desired, garnish with jalapeño pepper slices. Keep still. 4. Cover. Depending on your slow cooker, simmer on low for 5-8 hours. Check the meat for tenderness after five hours. Alternatively, heat the food until it is soft but not dry.

Per Serving: Calories 206; Total Fat 7g; Saturated Fat 2g; Sodium 122mg; Carbs 4g; Fiber 1g; Sugar 2g; Protein 30g

Roasted Rump and Vegetables Stew

Prep Time: 20 minutes | Cook Time: 10-12 hours | Serves: 8

1½ lbs. small potatoes (about 10), or medium potatoes (about 4), halved, unpeeled
2 medium carrots, cubed
1 small onion, sliced
10-oz. pkg. frozen lima beans
1 bay leaf
2 tbsps. quick-cooking tapioca

2-2½ lb. boneless beef round rump, round tip, or pot roast, trimmed of fat
2 tbsps. canola oil
10¾-oz. can condensed vegetable beef soup
¼ cup water
¼ tsp. pepper

1. In the slow cooker, add the potatoes, carrots, and onions. Bay leaf and frozen beans are added. Add a sprinkle of tapioca. 2. Roast is seared in oil in a pan from both sides. Put it on top of the slow cooker's veggies. 3. Mix the soup, water, and pepper together. Add to the roast. 4. Cover. Cook for 10–12 hours on low or 6–8 hours on high. 5. Before serving, throw away the bay leaf.

Per Serving: Calories 418; Total Fat 10g; Saturated Fat 3g; Sodium 336mg; Carbs 37g; Fiber 6g; Sugar 5g; Protein 42g

Chapter 6 Stew, Soups, Salads, and Sandwiches Recipes

Herbed Vegetables Pasta

Prep time: 10 minutes | Cook time: 25 minutes | Serves: 12

1 tablespoon extra-virgin olive oil
1 large onion, chopped
3 cloves garlic, crushed
2 medium carrots, sliced
2 medium zucchini, sliced
2 tablespoons finely chopped fresh basil

2 teaspoons finely chopped fresh oregano
Two 14.5-ounce cans unsalted tomatoes with liquid
Two 15-ounce cans low-sodium white cannellini or navy beans, drained and rinsed
¾ pound whole-wheat uncooked rigatoni or shell pasta

1. In a saucepan, sauté the onion and garlic in hot oil for 5 minutes. 2. Add the carrots, zucchini, basil, oregano, tomatoes with their liquid, and beans. Cook until veggies are tender, about 15–17 minutes. 3. In a separate saucepan, cook the pasta according to package directions (without adding salt). Add the pasta to the soup, and mix thoroughly. Serve warm with crusty bread.
Per Serving: Calories 210; Total Fat 2g; Saturated Fat 0.3g; Sodium 25mg; Carbs 40g; Fiber 8g; Sugar 6g; Protein 9g

Clam and Veggie Chowder

Prep time: 10 minutes | Cook time: 1 ½ hours | Serves: 8

3 carrots, coarsely chopped
3 potatoes, coarsely chopped
4 celery stalks, coarsely chopped
2½ cups minced clams, drained

2 cups canned tomatoes, slightly crushed
½ teaspoon dried thyme
Ground black pepper

1. Add all ingredients to a stockpot. Cover and let simmer for 1½ hours. Serve hot.
Per Serving: Calories 150; Total Fat 1g; Saturated Fat 0.1g; Sodium 180mg; Carbs 21g; Fiber 3g; Sugar 4g; Protein 15g

Shrimp and Brown Rice

Prep time: 10 minutes | Cook time: 40 minutes | Serves: 4

2 cups low-sodium canned tomatoes, undrained
¼ cup chopped green bell pepper
1 medium onion, chopped
1 cup cooked brown rice
½ cup low-sodium chicken broth

1 medium garlic clove, minced
Dash hot pepper sauce
Freshly ground black pepper
12 ounces precooked fresh jumbo shrimp

1. Place all the ingredients instead of the shrimp in a large stockpot and bring to a boil. Manage simmer on low heat for 25–30 minutes. 2. Add the shrimp, cover, and simmer for 5–10 minutes or until the shrimp is thoroughly heated. Serve hot.
Per Serving: Calories 190; Total Fat 1g; Saturated Fat 0.2g; Sodium 125mg; Carbs 22g; Fiber 3g; Sugar 5g; Protein 24g

Black Bean Soup

Prep time: 5 minutes | Cook time: 1 hour 10 minutes | Serves: 6

1½ cups plus 2 teaspoons low-sodium chicken broth, divided
1 teaspoon extra-virgin olive oil
3 garlic cloves, minced
1 yellow onion, minced
1 teaspoon minced fresh oregano

1 teaspoon cumin
1 teaspoon chili powder or ½ teaspoon cayenne pepper
1 red bell pepper, chopped
1 carrot, coarsely chopped
3 cups cooked black beans
½ cup dry red wine

1. In a large pot, heat 2 teaspoons of the chicken broth and the olive oil. Sauté the garlic, onion, for 3 minutes. Add the oregano with cumin seeds, and chili powder; stir for another minute. Add the red pepper and carrot. 2. Puree 1½ cups of the black beans in a blender or food processor. Add the pureed beans, the remaining 1½ cups of whole black beans, the remaining 1½ cups of chicken broth, and the red wine to the stockpot. Simmer 1 hour. 3. Taste before serving; add additional spices if you like.

Per Serving: Calories 160; Total Fat 1.5g; Saturated Fat 0.3g; Sodium 55mg; Carbs 26g; Fiber 9g; Sugar 5g; Protein 10g

Herbed Cherry Tomato Salad

Prep time: 7 minutes | Cook time: 0 minutes | Serves: 2 to 4

1-pint cherry tomatoes, halved
1 bunch fresh parsley, leaves only
1 cup cilantro, leaves only (stems discarded)
¼ cup fresh dill

1 teaspoon sumac (optional)
2 tablespoons extra-virgin olive oil
Kosher salt
Freshly ground black pepper

1. In a medium bowl, carefully toss together the tomatoes, parsley, cilantro, dill, sumac (if using), olive oil, and salt, pepper to taste.

Per Serving: Calories 161; Total Fat 14g; Saturated Fat 3g; Sodium 322mg; Carbs 8g; Fiber 3g; Sugar 5g; Protein 3g

Spicy Turkey Chili

Prep time: 10 minutes | Cook time: 50 minutes | Serves: 6

2 onions, chopped
2 garlic cloves, minced
½ cup green bell pepper
1 tablespoon olive oil
1-pound lean ground turkey meat
2 cups cooked kidney beans

2 cups tomatoes with liquid
1 cup low-sodium chicken broth
2 tablespoon chili powder
2 teaspoons cumin
Freshly ground black pepper

1. In a saucepan, sauté the onion, garlic, green pepper in the hot oil for 10 minutes. Add the turkey meat in it, and sauté until the turkey is cooked, about 5–10 minutes. 2 Add all the remaining ingredients, boil it, manage simmer on low heat uncovered for 30 minutes.

Per Serving: Calories 240; Total Fat 5g; Saturated Fat 0.9g; Sodium 200mg; Carbs 24g; Fiber 7g; Sugar 5g; Protein 27g

Creamy Beans Soup

Prep time: 5 minutes | Cook time: 2 ½ hours | Serves: 6

¼ cup chopped onion
1 garlic clove, minced
2 tablespoons extra-virgin olive oil
½ pound dried great northern, white navy, or cannellini beans, soaked in boiling water for 1 hour and drained
2 quarts water

2 bay leaves
1 teaspoon dried basil
teaspoon salt
teaspoon freshly ground black pepper
2 medium scallions, chopped
2 tablespoons minced fresh parsley

1. In a saucepan, sauté the onion and garlic in the oil for 5 minutes. Add the beans, water, bay leaves, and basil; stir well. Boil the mix, lower the heat, cover, and let simmer. 2. Continue to cook the soup for 1–1½ hours or until the beans are tender. Add water (if necessary), salt, and pepper; mix well. 3. Remove and discard the bay leaves. In a food processor, puree the mixture. Return the soup to the saucepan and serve hot. Garnish with scallions and parsley.
Per Serving: Calories 150; Total Fat 5g; Saturated Fat 0.8g; Sodium 25mg; Carbs 20g; Fiber 7g; Sugar 2g; Protein 8g

Minty Citrus Avocado Salad

Prep time: 10 minutes | Cook time: 0 minutes | Serves: 2

4 cups salad greens
1 grapefruit, peeled and segmented
1 orange, peeled and segmented
2 tablespoons minced red onion
¼ cup fresh mint leaves, torn

3 tablespoons Lemon Vinaigrette Dressing or store-bought
1 avocado, thinly sliced
¼ cup Stovetop Granola (optional)

1. In a bowl, toss the salad greens, grapefruit, orange, red onion, mint, and dressing. 2. Place the salad on a plate with the slices of avocado and a sprinkling of granola.
Per Serving: Calories 364; Total Fat 26g; Saturated Fat 2g; Sodium 125mg; Carbs 32g; Fiber 9g; Sugar 5g; Protein 6g

Cheese Baby Spinach and Strawberries Salad

Prep time: 7 minutes | Cook time: 0 minutes | Serves: 2 to 4

8 cups packed fresh baby spinach
16 strawberries, quartered
4 ounces goat cheese, crumbled
¼ cup chopped toasted almonds

2 tablespoons Lemon Vinaigrette Dressing or store-bought
Kosher salt
Freshly ground black pepper

1. In a bowl, gently toss together the spinach, strawberries, goat cheese, and almonds. Drizzle the salad with the vinaigrette and season with salt and pepper to taste. 2. Store any leftovers in an airtight container in the refrigerator for up to 3 days, but the salad is best consumed on the day it is dressed.
Per Serving: Calories 516; Total Fat 39g; Saturated Fat 0.6g; Sodium 455mg; Carbs 21g; Fiber 8g; Sugar 2g; Protein 25g

Asparagus Salad with Chile-Lime Dressing

Prep time: 15 minutes | Cook time: 0 minutes | Serves: 2 to 4

1 bunch asparagus, woody ends trimmed and stalks peeled into ribbons

12 ounces leftover rotisserie chicken (optional)

2 cups shredded cabbage

1 cup arugula

1 bunch (about 8) radishes, thinly sliced

½ cup mint, stemmed and finely sliced

3 scallions, finely sliced

¼ to ½ cup Chile-Lime Dressing or store-bought

⅓ cup chopped, roasted (unsalted) peanuts

Pickled Red Onions (optional)

1. Combine the asparagus ribbons, chicken (if using), cabbage, arugula, radishes, mint, and scallions in a large bowl. Pour dressing and toss to combine with your hands or tongs. 2. Place the salad on a large serving plate and garnish it with the chopped peanuts, pickled red onions, and more chopped mint if you like.

Per Serving: Calories 391; Total Fat 30g; Saturated Fat 5g; Sodium 312mg; Carbs 25g; Fiber 10g; Sugar 6g; Protein 13g

Cucumber, Beans, and Corn Salad

Prep Time: 10 minutes | Cook Time: 2 minutes | Serves: 4

3 cups diced cucumber

1 (15-ounce) can low-sodium dark red kidney beans, drained and rinsed

2 avocados, diced

1½ cups diced tomatoes

1 cup cooked corn

¾ cup sliced red onion

1 tablespoon extra-virgin olive oil

1 tablespoon apple cider vinegar

1. Cucumber, kidney beans, avocados, tomatoes, corn, onion, olive oil, and vinegar should all be combined in a large dish. Stir to mix well and serve.

Per Serving: Calories 453; Total Fat 19g; Saturated Fat 2g; Sodium 198mg; Carbs 63g; Fiber 17g; Sugar 6g; Protein 13g

Lemon Cauliflower and Pomegranate Arils Salad

Prep time: 20 minutes | Cook time: 5 minutes | Serves: 4-6

⅓ cup extra-virgin olive oil, divided

4 cups grated cauliflower

Juice of 1 lemon

¼ red onion, minced

4 large tomatoes, diced

3 large bunches flat-leaf parsley, chopped

1 large bunch mint, chopped

½ cup pomegranate arils

Kosher salt

Freshly ground black pepper

1. In a skillet, heat extra-virgin olive oil. When it's hot, add the cauliflower and sauté for 3 to 5 minutes or until it starts to crisp. Allow the cauliflower to cool while you prep the remaining ingredients. 2. In a large bowl, combine the remaining extra-virgin olive oil with the lemon juice and red onion. Mix well, then mix in the tomatoes, parsley, mint, and pomegranate arils. 3. After the cauliflower cools, 5 to 7 minutes, add it to the bowl with the other ingredients. Spice with salt and pepper and serve.

Per Serving: Calories 270; Total Fat 19g; Saturated Fat 3g; Sodium 388mg; Carbs 22g; Fiber 8g; Sugar 6g; Protein 7g

Cheese Brussels Sprouts Salad with Poppy Seed Dressing

Prep time: 20 minutes | Cook time: 0 minutes | Serves: 4-6

1 pound Brussels sprouts, shaved
1 bunch kale, thinly shredded
4 scallions, thinly sliced
4 ounces shredded Romano cheese

Poppy Seed Dressing or store-bought
Kosher salt
Freshly ground black pepper

1. In a bowl, toss the Brussels sprouts, kale, scallions, and Romano cheese. 2. Add the dressing to the greens and toss to combine. Season with salt and pepper to taste.

Per Serving: Calories 251; Total Fat 12g; Saturated Fat 1g; Sodium 122mg; Carbs 23g; Fiber 6g; Sugar 3g; Protein 14g

Feta Quinoa and Cucumber Salad

Prep time: 10 minutes | Cook time: 15 minutes | Serves: 2

1 cup quinoa, rinsed
2 cups water
Kosher salt
Freshly ground black pepper
1 bunch fresh parsley, minced

1 medium cucumber, cut into ¼-inch dice
¼ cup minced red onion
2 tablespoons toasted sesame seeds
¼ to ½ cup Tahini Dressing or store-bought
4 ounces crumbled feta

1. In a saucepan, mix the quinoa with the water and a pinch each of salt and pepper. Boil it over medium-high heat, then decrease to a gentle simmer and allow to cook for 10-15 minutes, until the quinoa absorbed all water. Remove the pot from the heat, cover, and allow to rest. 2. In a bowl, mix the parsley, cucumber, red onion, sesame seeds, and dressing. 3. Add the cooked quinoa to the bowl with the other ingredients. Toss well to coat evenly and spice with salt and pepper. 4. Top the salad with feta and serve. 5. Store any leftovers in an airtight container in the refrigerator for 3 to 5 days.

Per Serving: Calories 653; Total Fat 27g; Saturated Fat 6g; Sodium 633mg; Carbs 78g; Fiber 13g; Sugar 14g; Protein 25g

Herbed Bulgur and Apple Salad

Prep time: 10 minutes | Cook time: 15 minutes | Serves: 2

2 cups water
1 cup bulgur
1 teaspoon dried thyme
2 tablespoons extra-virgin olive oil
2 teaspoons cider vinegar

Kosher salt
Freshly ground black pepper
6 kale leaves, shredded
1 small apple, cored and diced
3 tablespoons sliced, toasted almonds

1. In a saucepan, boil water over high heat and remove it from the heat. Add the bulgur and thyme, cover, and allow the grain to rest for 7 to 15 minutes or until cooked through. 2. In a bowl, whisk the extra-virgin olive oil and cider vinegar with a pinch of salt and pepper. Add the cooked bulgur, kale, apple, and almonds to the dressing and toss to combine. Adjust the seasonings as desired.

Per Serving: Calories 550; Total Fat 20g; Saturated Fat 3g; Sodium 321mg; Carbs 82g; Fiber 21g; Sugar 13g; Protein 15g

Cheese Farro and Beets Bowl

Prep time: 1 minutes | Cook time: 20 minutes | Serves: 2

3 cups water
1 cup farro, rinsed
2 tablespoons extra-virgin olive oil
1 tablespoon honey
3 tablespoons cider vinegar
Pinch freshly ground black pepper

4 small cooked beets, sliced
1 pear, cored and diced
6 cups mixed greens
⅓ cup pumpkin seeds, roasted
¼ cup ricotta cheese

1. In a saucepan, stir the water and farro over high heat and bring to a boil. Reduce the heat and manage simmer until the farro is tender, 15 to 20 minutes. Drain and rinse the farro under cold running water until cool. Set aside. 2. In a bowl, Mix the oil with honey, and vinegar. Season with black pepper. 3. Evenly divide the farro between two bowls. Top each with the beets, pear, greens, pumpkin seeds, and ricotta. Drizzle the bowls with the dressing before serving and adjust the seasonings as desired.
Per Serving: Calories 779; Total Fat 29g; Saturated Fat 0.1g; Sodium 322mg; Carbs 108g; Fiber 15g; Sugar 20g; Protein 26g

Grilled Romaine with White Beans

Prep time: 5 minutes | Cook time: 8 minutes | Serves: 4-6

3 tablespoons extra-virgin olive oil, divided
2 large heads romaine lettuce, halved lengthwise
2 tablespoons white miso

1 tablespoon water, plus more as needed
1 (15-ounce) can white beans
½ cup chopped fresh parsley

1. Preheat the grill. 2. Drizzle 2 tablespoons of extra-virgin olive oil over the cut sides of the romaine lettuce. 3. In a medium bowl, whisk the remaining 1 tablespoon of extra-virgin olive oil with the white miso and about 1 tablespoon of water. Add the white beans and parsley to the bowl, stir, adjust the seasonings as desired, and set aside. 4. When the grill is hot, put the romaine on the grill and cook for 1 to 2 minutes on each side or until lightly charred with grill marks. Remove the lettuce from the grill and repeat with remaining lettuce halves. Set the lettuce aside on a platter or individual plates and top with the beans. 5. Serve.
Per Serving: Calories 291; Total Fat 12g; Saturated Fat 0.3g; Sodium 258mg; Carbs 38g; Fiber 14g; Sugar 15g; Protein 14g

Chicken Almonds Salad

Prep time: 10 minutes | Cook time: 0 minutes | Serves: 4

1 cup plain Greek yogurt
2 tablespoons minced shallots
1 teaspoon ground coriander
1 teaspoon Dijon mustard (optional)
1 tablespoon freshly squeezed lemon juice
¼ teaspoon cayenne pepper

12 ounces cooked rotisserie chicken, shredded
2 cups chopped celery with the leaves
¼ cup slivered almonds, toasted
¼ cup thinly sliced dried apricots
1 bunch fresh parsley, chopped

1. In a bowl, add the yogurt along with shallots, coriander, mustard (if using), lemon juice, and cayenne until well combined. 2. Add the chicken, celery, almonds, apricots, and parsley. 3. Serve on your food of choice.
Per Serving: Calories 288; Total Fat 16g; Saturated Fat 3g; Sodium 333mg; Carbs 12g; Fiber 3g; Sugar 4g; Protein 25g

Chickpea Fattoush Salad with Pitas

Prep time: 15 minutes | Cook time: 5 minutes | Serves: 4

2 tablespoons extra-virgin olive oil
2 pitas, torn into bite-size pieces
1 (15-ounce) can chickpeas, rinsed and drained
1 head romaine lettuce, cut into bite-size pieces
1 cucumber, diced
½ pint cherry tomatoes, halved

8 radishes, thinly sliced
1 bunch fresh parsley, chopped
1 cup mint, chopped
½ teaspoon sumac (optional)
½ cup Lemon Vinaigrette Dressing or store-bought

1. Heat the extra-virgin olive oil and sauté the pita bread until toasted and crisp, about 3 minutes. Remove the skillet from the heat and transfer the pita bread to a medium bowl. 2. Add the chickpeas, romaine, cucumber, tomatoes, radishes, parsley, mint, and sumac (if using) to the medium bowl. Add the dressing and toss to combine. Serve. 3. Store any leftovers in an airtight container in the refrigerator for up to 3 days.

Per Serving: Calories 466; Total Fat 30g; Saturated Fat 0.5g; Sodium 369mg; Carbs 42g; Fiber 10g; Sugar 11g; Protein 11g

Roasted Carrot with Quinoa & Pistachios

Prep time: 10 minutes | Cook time: 20 minutes | Serves: 4

4 large carrots, cut into ⅛-inch-thick rounds
4 tablespoons oil (olive, safflower, or grapeseed), divided
2 teaspoons paprika
1 teaspoon turmeric
2 teaspoons ground cumin

2 cups water
1 cup quinoa, rinsed
½ cup shelled pistachios, toasted
4 ounces goat cheese
12 ounces salad greens

1. Preheat the oven to 400°F temp setting. Manage a baking sheet with parchment paper. 2. In a large bowl, toss together the carrots, 2 tablespoons of oil, the paprika, turmeric, and cumin until the carrots are well coated. Spread them evenly on the prepared baking sheet and roast until tender, 15 to 17 minutes. 3. In a saucepan, mix the water and quinoa over high heat. Boil it, lower the heat and simmer until tender, about 15 minutes. 4. Transfer the roasted carrots to a large bowl and add the cooked quinoa, remaining 2 tablespoons of oil, the pistachios, and goat cheese and toss to combine. 5. Evenly divide the greens among four plates and top with the carrot mixture. Serve. 6. Store any leftovers in an airtight container in the refrigerator for up to 2 days.

Per Serving: Calories 527; Total Fat 31g; Saturated Fat 10g; Sodium 257mg; Carbs 48g; Fiber 10g; Sugar 11g; Protein 17g

Homemade Chicken and Cucumber Sandwiches

Prep Time: 10 minutes | Cook Time: 5 minutes | Serves: 3

3 tablespoons red pepper hummus
3 slices 100% whole-wheat bread, toasted
¾ cup cucumber slices
3 cups arugula or baby kale

¼ cup sliced red onion
1 cup shredded rotisserie chicken
Oregano, for garnish (optional)

1. Each piece of toasted bread should have 1 tablespoon of hummus spread on it. 2. On each slice of bread, arrange a third of the cucumber, arugula, onion, and chicken. Oregano is for garnishing (if using).

Per Serving: Calories 262; Total Fat 13g; Saturated Fat 3g; Sodium 183mg; Carbs 16g; Fiber 2g; Sugar 1g; Protein 18g

Feta Chicken, Cantaloupe and Kale Salad

Prep Time: 10 minutes | Cook Time: 2 minutes |Serves: 3

For the Salad
cups chopped kale, packed
1½ cups diced cantaloupe
1½ cups shredded rotisserie chicken
½ cup sliced almonds
¼ cup crumbled feta

For the Dressing
2 teaspoons honey
2 tablespoons extra-virgin olive oil
2 teaspoons apple cider vinegar or freshly squeezed lemon juice

To make the salad: 1. Three parts of kale should be divided. On each serving, arrange a third of the cantaloupe, chicken, almonds, and feta. 2. Each salad serving should have some of the dressing drizzled on it. Serve right away.
To make the dressing: In a small bowl, whisk together the honey, olive oil, and vinegar.
Per Serving: Calories 256; Total Fat 16g; Saturated Fat 5g; Sodium 215mg; Carbs 10g; Fiber 1g; Sugar 9g; Protein 16g

Chicken, Spinach and Strawberries Salad

Prep Time: 10 minutes | Cook Time: 5 minutes |Serves: 4

For the Salad
2 cups baby spinach
2 cups shredded rotisserie chicken
½ cup sliced strawberries or other berries
½ cup sliced almonds
1 avocado, sliced

¼ cup crumbled feta (optional)
For the Dressing
2 tablespoons extra-virgin olive oil
2 teaspoons honey
2 teaspoons balsamic vinegar

To make the salad: 1. Combine the spinach, chicken, strawberries, and almonds in a big bowl. 2. Then, give the salad a quick toss after adding the dressing. 3. Top each of the four equal servings with a slice of avocado and a spoonful of crumbled feta cheese (if using).
To Make the dressing: 1. In a small bowl, whisk together the olive oil, honey, and balsamic vinegar.
Per Serving: Calories 1155; Total Fat 82g; Saturated Fat 22g; Sodium 520mg; Carbs 11g; Fiber 5g; Sugar 5g; Protein 90g

Healthy Egg and Spinach Sandwiches

Prep Time: 10 minutes | Cook Time: 5 minutes |Serves: 4

8 large hardboiled eggs
3 tablespoons plain low-fat Greek yogurt
1 tablespoon mustard
½ teaspoon freshly ground black pepper

1 teaspoon chopped fresh chives
4 slices 100% whole-wheat bread
2 cups fresh spinach, loosely packed

1. Cut the eggs in half after peeling them. 2. With a fork, mash the eggs in a big bowl, leaving some lumps.
Mix in the chives, mustard, yogurt, and pepper. 3. Place one piece of bread, one-fourth of the egg salad, and one spinach leaf on each serving.
Per Serving: Calories 222; Total Fat 10g; Saturated Fat 3g; Sodium 246mg; Carbs 23g; Fiber 3g; Sugar 1g; Protein 10g

Roasted Tomatoes and Cheese Sandwich

Prep time: 5 minutes | Cook time: 15 minutes | Serves: 2

3 tomatoes, cut into eighths
2 tablespoons extra-virgin olive oil, divided
1 tablespoon balsamic vinegar
2 garlic cloves, minced
Pinch kosher salt

Pinch freshly ground black pepper
½ cup ricotta cheese
2 slices whole-grain bread
2 tablespoons chopped fresh basil
4 cups arugula

1. Preheat the oven to 450°F. Manage a baking sheet with parchment paper. 2. In a medium-sized bowl, toss the tomatoes with 1 tablespoon of extra-virgin olive oil, the vinegar, garlic, salt, and pepper. 3. Spread the tomatoes on the baking sheet and bake for 15 minutes. 4. Meanwhile, place the ricotta in the bowl of a food processor and, while it is running, add the remaining 1 tablespoon of extra-virgin olive oil in a thin stream. Taste and adjust the seasonings as needed. Whisk the ricotta and extra-virgin olive oil in a medium bowl. 5. Toast the bread and divide the ricotta between the slices, spreading it out evenly. Top the ricotta with the tomatoes and garnish with chopped basil. 6. Serve with the greens on the side.
Per Serving: Calories 375; Total Fat 22g; Saturated Fat 10g; Sodium 231mg; Carbs 34g; Fiber 6g; Sugar 7g; Protein 13g

Mushroom-Cauliflower Lettuce Wraps

Prep time: 10 minutes | Cook time: 20 minutes | Serves: 2-4

1½ tablespoons sesame oil
½ yellow onion, chopped
8 ounces mushrooms, thinly sliced
4 garlic cloves, minced
1½ tablespoons low-sodium soy sauce or tamari
4 teaspoons rice wine vinegar

5 ounces water chestnuts, drained and liquid reserved
2½ cups Cauliflower Rice
½ cup coarsely chopped cashews
4 large green leaf lettuce leaves
2 scallions, thinly sliced (optional)
1 cup chopped cilantro (optional)

1. Heat the sesame oil and sauté the onion until translucent, about 3 minutes. Add the mushrooms, garlic, tamari, vinegar, and water chestnuts to the skillet. Cover and cook until the mushrooms are softened, about 5 minutes. 2. Add the cauliflower and cashews and mix well. Cover and cook for 2 minutes. 3. Adjust the seasonings as desired and evenly divide the cauliflower mixture among the lettuce leaves. 4. Serve garnished with scallions (if using) and cilantro (if using).
Per Serving: Calories 413; Total Fat 25g; Saturated Fat 8g; Sodium 452mg; Carbs 38g; Fiber 9g; Sugar 9g; Protein 17g

Feta Steak and Spinach Salad

Prep Time: 10 minutes | Cook Time: 15 minutes |Serves: 4

4 ounces homemade sofrito or low-sodium vegetable broth
2 (4-ounce) flank steaks
8 cups fresh spinach, loosely packed
½ cup sliced red onion

2 cups diced tomato
2 avocados, diced
2 cups diced cucumber
⅓ cup crumbled feta

1. A big skillet should be heated slowly. Pour the sofrito in once it is heated, then add the steaks and cover. For 8 to 12 minutes, cook. 2. Divide the spinach into four equal sections as you wait. Addt a quarter of each of the onion, tomato, avocado, and cucumber to the top of each serving. 3. Before slicing, take the steak out of the griddle and let it rest for about 2 minutes. Top each serving with a quarter of the feta and the meat.
Per Serving: Calories 407; Total Fat 24g; Saturated Fat 6g; Sodium 335mg; Carbs 16g; Fiber 9g; Sugar 4g; Protein 32g

Refreshing Avocado, Tomato, and Cucumber Salad

Prep Time: 10 minutes | Cook Time: 2 minutes |Serves: 4

1 cup cherry tomatoes, halved
1 large cucumber, chopped
1 small red onion, thinly sliced
1 avocado, diced
2 tablespoons chopped fresh dill

2 tablespoons extra-virgin olive oil
Juice of 1 lemon
¼ teaspoon salt
¼ teaspoon freshly ground black pepper

1. Combine the tomatoes, cucumber, onion, avocado, and dill in a large mixing basin. 2. Add the oil, lemon juice, salt, and pepper in a bowl and stir to combine. 3. Dress the veggies by drizzling the dressing over them and mixing. Serve.
Per Serving: Calories 151; Total Fat 12.3g; Saturated Fat 5g; Sodium 123mg; Carbs 11g; Fiber 4.2g; Sugar 4g; Protein 2.14g

Easy Cabbage and Carrot Salad

Prep Time: 15 minutes | Cook Time: 2 minutes |Serves: 6

2 cups finely chopped green cabbage
2 cups finely chopped red cabbage
2 cups grated carrots
3 scallions, both white and green parts, sliced
2 tablespoons extra-virgin olive oil

2 tablespoons rice vinegar
1 teaspoon honey
1 garlic clove, minced
¼ teaspoon salt

1. Combine the green and red cabbage, carrots, and onions in a large bowl. 2. Combine the oil, vinegar, honey, garlic, and salt in a small bowl. 3. Drop the dressing over the vegetables, then toss to incorporate. 4. Either serve right away, or cover and refrigerate for several hours.
Per Serving: Calories 80; Total Fat 5g; Saturated Fat 1g; Sodium 127mg; Carbs 10g; Fiber 6g; Sugar 3g; Protein 1.4g

Sweet Potatoes & Greens Salad with Blackberry Vinaigrette

Prep Time: 15 minutes | Cook Time: 20 minutes |Serves: 4

For the Vinaigrette:
1 pint blackberries
2 tablespoons red wine vinegar
1 tablespoon honey
3 tablespoons extra-virgin olive oil
¼ teaspoon salt
Freshly ground black pepper

For the Salad:
1 sweet potato, cubed
1 teaspoon extra-virgin olive oil
2 cups salad greens (baby spinach, spicy greens, romaine)
½ red onion, sliced
¼ cup crumbled goat cheese

To make the vinaigrette: The blackberries, vinegar, honey, oil, salt, and pepper should all be combined in a blender jar and blended until smooth. Set aside. To make the salad: 1. Set the oven to 425°F. Use parchment paper to cover a baking sheet. 2. Combine the olive oil and sweet potato in a medium mixing dish. When the food is soft, transfer to the prepared baking sheet and roast for 20 minutes, stirring halfway through. Remove and let cool briefly. 3. Combine the greens, red onion, and cooled sweet potato in a large bowl and top with vinaigrette. Per serving, sprinkle 1 tablespoon of goat cheese on top.
Per Serving: Calories 196; Total Fat 12.3g; Saturated Fat 5g; Sodium 203mg; Carbs 21g; Fiber 10.2g; Sugar 6g; Protein 4g

Flavorful Chicken and Grape Sandwiches

Prep Time: 10 minutes | Cook Time: 15 minutes |Serves: 4

Avocado oil cooking spray
2 (4-ounce) boneless, skinless chicken breasts
⅛ teaspoon freshly ground black pepper
1½ tablespoons plain low-fat Greek yogurt

¼ cup halved purple seedless grapes
¼ cup chopped pecans
2 tablespoons chopped celery
4 sandwich thins, 100% whole-wheat

1. A small skillet should be heated slowly. Spray cooking spray on the cooking surface once it is heated. 2. Season the chicken with the pepper. Cook the chicken for 6 minutes in the skillet. After flipping, heat for an another 3 to 5 minutes, or until well cooked. 3. The chicken should be taken out of the skillet and given five minutes to cool. Shred or chop the chicken. 4. Combine the grapes, pecans, celery, and yogurt with the chicken. The sandwich thins should be divided into a top and a bottom. 5. Divide the chicken salad into four equal halves, place a portion on each of the sandwich thins' bottom half, then top with the remaining halves.

Per Serving: Calories 235; Total Fat 10g; Saturated Fat 2g; Sodium 44mg; Carbs 21g; Fiber 4g; Sugar 2g; Protein 15g

Chicken and Tomato Sandwiches

Prep Time: 5 minutes | Cook Time: 5 minutes |Serves: 4

For the Dressing:
4 tablespoons plain low-fat Greek yogurt
4 teaspoons Dijon mustard
4 teaspoons freshly squeezed lemon juice
4 teaspoons shredded Parmesan cheese
¼ teaspoon freshly ground black pepper
⅛ teaspoon garlic powder

For the Sandwiches:
2 cups shredded rotisserie chicken
1½ cups chopped romaine lettuce
12 cherry tomatoes, halved
4 sandwich thins, 100% whole-wheat
¼ cup thinly sliced red onion (optional)

To make the dressing: Mix the yogurt, mustard, lemon juice, Parmesan cheese, black pepper, and garlic powder in a small bowl.To make the sandwiches: 1. Combine the chicken, lettuce, and tomatoes in a big bowl. When the dressing is added, mix it in well. Four equal amounts of the filling should be taken. 2. Cut the thin sandwich slices in half, top and bottom, for each. Each bottom half should have a piece of filling on it. 3. The top halves should then be placed on top.

Per Serving: Calories 382; Total Fat 20g; Saturated Fat 6g; Sodium 206mg; Carbs 22g; Fiber 4g; Sugar 2g; Protein 28g

Cheese Pulled Pork Sandwiches

Prep Time: 5 minutes | Cook Time: 15 minutes |Serves: 4

Avocado oil cooking spray
8 ounces store-bought pulled pork
½ cup chopped green bell pepper

2 slices provolone cheese
4 sandwich thins, 100% whole-wheat
2½ tablespoons apricot jelly

1. As directed on the packaging, reheat the pulled pork. 2. Over medium-low heat, preheat a medium skillet. Spray cooking spray on the cooking surface once it is heated. 3. Cook the bell pepper for 5 minutes in a skillet. Transfer to a small bowl, then reserve. 4. While you wait, cut the sandwich thins in half to create a top and bottom and tear each piece of cheese into two strips. 5. Place the sandwich thins in the pan cut-side down and toast for 2 minutes on low heat. 6. Sandwich thins should be taken off of the skillet. Place one-quarter of the cheese, pulled pork, and pepper on top of each sandwich's bottom half after spreading one-quarter of the jelly on it. the thin top part of the sandwich to cover.

Per Serving: Calories 168; Total Fat 6g; Saturated Fat 3g; Sodium 502mg; Carbs 16g; Fiber 1g; Sugar 14g; Protein 11g

Garlicky Carrot and Kale Soup

Prep Time: 10 minutes | Cook Time: 15 minutes |Serves: 4

1 tablespoon extra-virgin olive oil
1 medium onion, chopped
2 carrots, finely chopped
3 garlic cloves, minced
4 cups low-sodium vegetable broth

1 (28-ounce) can crushed tomatoes
½ teaspoon dried oregano
¼ teaspoon dried basil
4 cups chopped baby kale leaves
¼ teaspoon salt

1. Over medium heat, warm the oil in a big saucepan. To the pan, add the onion and carrots. They should soften after 3 to 5 minutes of sautéing. 30 seconds later, add the garlic and continue to cook until fragrant. 2. Fill the saucepan with the tomatoes, oregano, basil, and vegetable broth. Bring to a boil. For five minutes, simmer over low heat. 3. Purée the soup in an immersion blender. 4. Add the greens and cook for a further three minutes. Use salt to season. Serve right away.

Per Serving: Calories 170; Total Fat 5g; Saturated Fat 1g; Sodium 603mg; Carbs 31g; Fiber 13.2g; Sugar 9g; Protein 6g

Beef and Pearl Barley Soup

Prep Time: 10 minutes | Cook Time: 1 hour and 20 minutes |Serves: 6

1-pound beef stew meat, cubed
¼ teaspoon salt
¼ teaspoon freshly ground black pepper
1 tablespoon extra-virgin olive oil
8 ounces sliced mushrooms
1 onion, chopped
2 carrots, chopped

3 celery stalks, chopped
6 garlic cloves, minced
½ teaspoon dried thyme
4 cups low-sodium beef broth
1 cup water
½ cup pearl barley

1. Salt and pepper should be used to season the meat. 2. Heat the oil in an Instant Pot over a high flame. Add the meat, then brown it completely. Take the meat out of the saucepan, then set it aside. 3. Add the mushrooms in the saucepan and heat for a couple of minutes, until they start to soften. The meat and the mushrooms should be removed and left aside. 4. Include the celery, onion, and carrots in the saucepan. Vegetables should be sautéed for 3 to 4 minutes until they start to soften. For another 30 seconds or so, add the garlic and continue to simmer until fragrant. 5. Add the thyme, beef broth, and water to the saucepan with the meat and mushrooms. Cook the food for 15 minutes using a high pressure setting. Let the pressure release naturally. 6. Open the Instant Pot and add the barley. Use the slow cooker function on the Instant Pot, affix the lid (vent open), and continue to cook for 1 hour until the barley is cooked through and tender. Serve.

Per Serving: Calories 245; Total Fat 9g; Saturated Fat 3g; Sodium 523mg; Carbs 19g; Fiber 3.2g; Sugar 4g; Protein 21.4g

Zucchini Soup with Roasted Chickpeas

Prep Time: 10 minutes | Cook Time: 20 minutes |Serves: 4

1 (15-ounce) can low-sodium chickpeas, drained and rinsed
1 teaspoon extra-virgin olive oil, plus 1 tablespoon
¼ teaspoon smoked paprika
Pinch salt, plus ½ teaspoon
3 medium zucchini, coarsely chopped

3 cups low-sodium vegetable broth
½ onion, diced
3 garlic cloves, minced
2 tablespoons plain low-fat Greek yogurt
Freshly ground black pepper

1. Set the oven to 425°F for preheating. Use parchment paper to cover a baking sheet. 2. Combine the chickpeas with 1 teaspoon of olive oil, the smoked paprika, and a dash of salt in a medium mixing bowl. Transfer to the prepared baking sheet, roast for 20 minutes, stirring once, until crispy. Place aside. 3. In the meantime, heat the final tablespoon of oil in a medium saucepan over medium heat. 4. Bring to a boil the broth, zucchini, onion, and garlic in the saucepan. Cook the zucchini and onion for approximately 20 minutes, then lower the heat to a simmer. 5. Purée the soup in a blender jar or with an immersion blender. Go back to the pot. 6. Stir in the yogurt and the final ½ teaspoon of salt and pepper. Serve topped with the roasted chickpeas.

Per Serving: Calories 180; Total Fat 7g; Saturated Fat 2g; Sodium 523mg; Carbs 25g; Fiber 7.2g; Sugar 7g; Protein 8g

Curry Coconut Carrot Soup

Prep Time: 10 minutes | Cook Time: 6 minutes |Serves: 6

1 tablespoon extra-virgin olive oil
1 small onion, coarsely chopped
2 celery stalks, coarsely chopped
1½ teaspoons curry powder
1 teaspoon ground cumin
1 teaspoon minced fresh ginger

6 medium carrots, roughly chopped
4 cups low-sodium vegetable broth
¼ teaspoon salt
1 cup canned coconut milk
¼ teaspoon freshly ground black pepper
1 tablespoon chopped fresh cilantro

1. Add the olive oil to an Instant Pot that is preheated to high. 2. Sauté the celery and onion for two to three minutes. Cook the curry powder, cumin, and ginger in the saucepan for approximately 30 seconds, or until aromatic. 3. Fill the container with the carrots, vegetable broth, and salt. Set the timer for 5 minutes on high, then close and seal. Allow the pressure to naturally decrease. 4. Carefully purée the soup in stages in a blender jar before returning it to the saucepan. 5. Stir in the pepper and coconut milk, then heat thoroughly. Add the cilantro on top before serving.

Per Serving: Calories 144; Total Fat 11g; Saturated Fat 5g; Sodium 323mg; Carbs 13g; Fiber 4.2g; Sugar 3g; Protein 3g

Lime Chicken Soup with Crispy Tortilla Strips

Prep Time: 10 minutes | Cook Time: 35 minutes |Serves: 4

1 tablespoon extra-virgin olive oil
1 onion, thinly sliced
1 garlic clove, minced
1 jalapeño pepper, diced
2 boneless, skinless chicken breasts
4 cups low-sodium chicken broth
1 roma tomato, diced

½ teaspoon salt
2 (6-inch) corn tortillas, cut into thin strips
Nonstick cooking spray
Juice of 1 lime
Minced fresh cilantro, for garnish
¼ cup shredded cheddar cheese, for garnish

1. Heat the oil to a medium-high temperature in a medium saucepan. After adding it, sauté the onion for 3 to 5 minutes, or until it starts to soften. About 1 minute further after adding the garlic and jalapeño, heat until aromatic. 2. Fill the saucepan with the chicken, chicken stock, tomato, and salt. Bring to a boil. The chicken breasts should be well cooked after 20 to 25 minutes of simmering over medium heat. Chicken should be taken out of the pot and placed aside. 3. Turn the broiler on high. Nonstick cooking spray the tortilla strips and toss to coat. 4. On a baking sheet, spread the ingredients in a single layer and broil for 3 to 5 minutes, turning once, or until crisp. 5. Use two forks to shred the chicken when it is cold enough to handle it, then add it back to the saucepan. 6. Add lime juice to the soup as a seasoning. Serve hot with cheese, tortilla strips, and cilantro as garnishes.
Per Serving: Calories 191; Total Fat 8g; Saturated Fat 5g; Sodium 488mg; Carbs 13.9g; Fiber 2.2g; Sugar 3g; Protein 21g

Chicken, Brussels Sprouts & Cranberries Salad

Prep Time: 10 minutes | Cook Time: 25 minutes |Serves: 4

For the Salad
(2-ounce) chicken tenders
Avocado oil cooking spray
2 slices turkey bacon
2 (9-ounce) packages shaved Brussels sprouts
2 hardboiled eggs, chopped

½ cup unsweetened dried cranberries
For the Dressing
3 tablespoons honey mustard
3 tablespoons extra-virgin olive oil
½ tablespoon freshly squeezed lemon juice

To make the salad: 1. Preheat the oven to 425ºF. 2. Cook the chicken tenders for 15 to 18 minutes after lightly spraying them with cooking spray and setting them on a baking sheet. 3. In the meantime, preheat a large skillet over low heat. Fry the bacon till crispy for 5 to 7 minutes while it's heated. When the bacon has finished cooking, gently take it from the pan and let it to cool and drain on a dish covered with paper towels. when it is cold enough to handle, crumble. 4. Chicken tenders should be cut into uniform pieces. Four equal quantities of Brussels sprouts should be cut up. Each serving should include one-quarter of the chopped eggs, bacon bits, dried cranberries, and two thinly sliced chicken tenders on top. 5. Pour a similar amount of dressing over each plate.
To make the dressing: In a small bowl, whisk together the mustard, olive oil, and lemon juice.
Per Serving: Calories 465; Total Fat 24g; Saturated Fat 4g; Sodium 411mg; Carbs 10g; Fiber 2g; Sugar 5g; Protein 28g

Kale Caesar Salad with Oat Croutons

Prep time: 8 minutes | Cook time: 15 minutes | Serves: 2 to 4

For the Oat Croutons:
½ cup rolled oats
1 tablespoon sunflower seeds
1 tablespoon chopped almonds
1 tablespoon canola oil
1 tablespoon honey
Pinch kosher salt

For the Salad:
1 bunch kale, cleaned, ribs removed, and chopped
1 bunch fresh parsley, leaves only
¼ cup Parmesan cheese
¼ to ½ cup Caesar Dressing or store-bought
1 lemon, cut into wedges (optional)

1. To make the oat croutons: Preheat the oven to 350°F temp setting. 2. In a small bowl, combine the oats, sunflower seeds, almonds, oil, honey, and a pinch of salt. Toss to coat evenly, then spread the mixture on a nonstick baking sheet. Bake for 12 to 15 minutes, then remove from the oven to cool on the baking sheet for 15 minutes. 3. To make the salad: In a bowl, toss the kale, parsley, and Parmesan cheese with the Caesar Dressing until all the leaves are coated. Place salad on plates. 4. Spread the croutons and serve. 5. If the dressing and oats are kept separately from the greens, then the salad and dressing will keep separately for 5 days in airtight containers in the refrigerator. The croutons will keep in an airtight container in the refrigerator for up to 1 month.
Per Serving: Calories 340; Total Fat 20g; Saturated Fat 5g; Sodium 302mg; Carbs 31g; Fiber 6g; Sugar 6g; Protein 12g

Basil Beans Salad

Prep Time: 10 minutes | Cook Time: 2 minutes |Serves: 8

1 (15-ounce) can low-sodium chickpeas, drained and rinsed
1 (15-ounce) can low-sodium kidney beans, drained and rinsed
1 (15-ounce) can low-sodium white beans, drained and rinsed
1 red bell pepper, seeded and finely chopped

¼ cup chopped scallions, both white and green parts
¼ cup finely chopped fresh basil
3 garlic cloves, minced
2 tablespoons extra-virgin olive oil
1 tablespoon red wine vinegar
1 teaspoon Dijon mustard
¼ teaspoon freshly ground black pepper

1. The chickpeas, kidney beans, white beans, bell pepper, scallions, basil, and garlic should all be combined in a large mixing basin. Gently blend by tossing. 2. Combine the olive oil, vinegar, mustard, and pepper in a small bowl. Include in the salad. 3. To give the flavors time to meld, cover and chill the dish for an hour before serving.
Per Serving: Calories 193; Total Fat 5g; Saturated Fat 1g; Sodium 243mg; Carbs 29g; Fiber 3.2g; Sugar 8g; Protein 10g

Smoky Tempeh and Carrot Rolls

Prep time: 10 minutes | Cook time: 10 minutes | Serves: 1

2 collard green leaves, washed
½ cup shredded carrots
1 teaspoon grated ginger (optional)
½ tablespoon white or yellow miso
½ tablespoon rice vinegar

½ tablespoon sesame oil
Nonstick cooking oil spray
4 ounces smoky tempeh, sliced
1 cup bean sprouts
4 radishes, thinly sliced

1. Fill a saucepan of water and bring it to a boil over high heat. Blanch the collard greens for 3 minutes, remove them from the water, and cool immediately under cold running water. Allow to dry and blot with a towel to remove excess water. 2. In a bowl, mix the carrots, ginger (if using), miso, vinegar, and sesame oil until well mixed. 3. Lightly grease a skillet and heat it over medium heat. Panfry the tempeh slices until crispy on each side, about 2 minutes per side. 4. Place the collard greens on a clean work surface and evenly divide the carrot mixture, tempeh, bean sprouts, and radishes between them. Fold over the end of each leaf, tuck one side under, and roll like a burrito. Serve. 5. Store any leftovers in an airtight container in the refrigerator for up to 2 days.

Per Serving: Calories 396; Total Fat 22g; Saturated Fat 12g; Sodium 536mg; Carbs 19g; Fiber 6g; Sugar 3g; Protein 31g

Delicious Cheese Chicken Spinach Sandwiches

Prep Time: 10 minutes | Cook Time: 15 minutes |Serves: 4

1 small yellow onion
Avocado oil cooking spray
2 cups shredded rotisserie chicken
1½ tablespoons unsalted butter

4 slices 100% whole-wheat bread
3 slices provolone or Swiss cheese
2 cups fresh spinach

1. Round the onion into ½ inch pieces. Do not split them apart; leave them whole. 2. Over medium-low heat, preheat a medium- or large skillet. Spray cooking spray on the cooking surface once it is heated. In the skillet, add the onions. When the onions are transparent, simmer with the lid on for 7 to 10 minutes. Take out of the skillet. 3. Meanwhile, butter one side of each slice of bread and shred the chicken. Cut each cheese slice into three strips. 4. Each slice of bread should have 2 or 3 cheese strips placed on the unbuttered side before being placed buttered side down on the pan. 5. On top of each slice of bread, arrange a quarter of the onion, spinach, and chicken. 6. Toast over low heat for two to three minutes.

Per Serving: Calories 442; Total Fat 28g; Saturated Fat 10g; Sodium 627mg; Carbs 18g; Fiber 2g; Sugar 2g; Protein 30g

Chapter 7 Dessert and Snack Recipes

Chocolate Avocado Mousse

Prep time: 10 minutes | Cook time: 0 minutes | Serves: 4

2 ripe avocados, pitted and peeled
¼ cup unsweetened cocoa powder
¼ cup full-fat coconut milk, plus extra as needed
2 to 4 tablespoons granulated sugar-free sweetener, such

as Swerve (optional)
2 teaspoons vanilla extract
½ teaspoon cinnamon (optional)
¼ teaspoon salt

1. In a blender, combine the avocados, cocoa powder, heavy cream, sweetener to taste (if using), vanilla, cinnamon (if using), and salt, and blend until smooth and creamy. If the mixture is too thick, add additional cream, 1 tablespoon at a time. 2. Serve immediately or store in an airtight container in the refrigerator for up to 2 days.
Per Serving: Calories 183; Total Fat 17g; Saturated Fat 5g; Sodium 158mg; Carbs 10g; Fiber 7g; Sugar 0g; Protein 3g

Raspberry-Chocolate Chia Pudding

Prep time: 10 minutes | Cook time: 15 minutes | Serves: 4

½ cup raspberries, fresh or frozen (thawed)
1 cup unsweetened almond milk
1 cup full-fat canned unsweetened coconut milk or heavy (whipping) cream

2 to 4 tablespoons granulated sugar-free sweetener, such as Swerve (optional)
½ cup chia seeds
¼ cup no-sugar-added chocolate protein powder

1. Put the raspberries in a large bowl and mash them well with a fork. Add the almond milk, coconut milk, and sweetener to taste (if using), and whisk until smooth. 2. Add the chia seeds along with protein powder, and whisk until well combined. 3. Divide the mixture evenly among 4 ramekins or small jars.
Per Serving: Calories 247; Total Fat 18g; Saturated Fat 10g; Sodium 95mg; Carbs 15g; Fiber 9g; Sugar 0g; Protein 11g

Lemon Avocado Dressing

Prep time: 10 minutes | Cook time: 0 minutes | Serves: 1 ½ cups

2 very ripe avocados, pitted and peeled
½ cup packed cilantro or parsley leaves
½ cup mayonnaise
Zest of 1 lemon
Juice of 1 lemon

1 teaspoon garlic powder
1 tablespoon dried chives or onion powder
1 teaspoon salt
¼ teaspoon freshly ground black pepper
Warm water, as needed

1. In a blender, blend the avocados, cilantro, mayonnaise, lemon zest and juice, garlic powder, dried chives, salt, and pepper until smooth. 2. The dressing will be thick. Add warm water, little at a time, blending after each addition to reach your desired consistency. A thicker dressing is great to use as a dipping sauce.
Per Serving: Calories 102; Total Fat 10g; Saturated Fat 2g; Sodium 257mg; Carbs 3g; Fiber 2g; Sugar 0g; Protein 1g

Minty Hot Chocolate

Prep time: 2 minutes | Cook time: 2 minutes | Serves: 1

1 cup unsweetened almond milk
¼ cup heavy (whipping) cream
1 teaspoon peppermint extract

2 tablespoons sugar-free chocolate chips, such as Lily's
2 tablespoons unsweetened cocoa powder
1 tablespoon granulated sweetener (optional)

1. In a microwave-safe mug, combine the almond milk, heavy cream, peppermint extract, and chocolate chips. Microwave on high for 90 seconds. 2. Remove and stir to blend the melted chips into the liquid. Add the cocoa powder and sweetener to taste (if using), and whisk with a fork until smooth. 3. Microwave for another 15 to 20 seconds. Whisk again and serve.

Per Serving: Calories 383; Total Fat 34g; Saturated Fat 20g; Sodium 191mg; Carbs 27g; Fiber 13g; Sugar 6g; Protein 7g

Strawberry Yogurt Pops

Prep time: 20 minutes | Cook time: 0 minutes | Serves: 5

12 ounces fresh or frozen (and thawed) s
trawberries, chopped
¼ cup plus 2 tablespoons granulated
sugar-free sweetener, such as Swerve, divided

1½ cups full-fat plain Greek yogurt
2 teaspoons vanilla extract
1½ cups heavy (whipping) cream

1. Combine the strawberries and ¼ cup of sweetener in a food processor and blend until pureed and smooth. 2. Place the mix to a bowl and mix in the yogurt and vanilla extract. 3. In bowl, using an electric mixer or by hand with a whisk, whip the cream with the remaining 2 tablespoons of sweetener until fluffy and stiff peaks have formed. 4. Fold the whipped cream into the yogurt-and-strawberry mixture until well combined. Freeze in ice-pop molds or transfer to a large airtight container and freeze until firm, 6 to 8 hours.

Per Serving: Calories 166; Total Fat 14g; Saturated Fat 9g; Sodium 24mg; Carbs 12g; Fiber 1g; Sugar 7g; Protein 5g

Tropical Fruit Salad

Prep time: 10 minutes | Cook time: 0 minutes | Serves: 8

2 cups pineapple chunks
2 kiwi fruits, peeled and sliced
1 mango, peeled and chopped

¼ cup canned light coconut milk
1 tablespoon freshly squeezed lime juice
1 tablespoon honey

1. In a bowl, toss the pineapple, kiwi, and mango. 2. In a small bowl, combine the coconut milk, lime juice, and honey, stirring until the honey dissolves. Pour over the fruits, and coat. Serve immediately or refrigerate in an airtight container for up to 3 days

Per Serving: Calories 70; Total Fat 1g; Saturated Fat 0g; Sodium 2mg; Carbs 17g; Fiber 2g; Sugar 14g; Protein 1g

Homemade Omega-3 Crackers

Prep time: 20 minutes | Cook time: 15 minutes | Serves: 6-8

1 cup almond flour
1 tablespoon flaxseed
1 tablespoon chia seed
1 tablespoon cumin seed (optional)

½ teaspoon salt
¼ teaspoon baking soda
1 large egg, beaten
1 tablespoon extra-virgin olive oil

1. Preheat the oven to 350°F temp setting. 2. In a large bowl, combine the almond flour, flaxseed, chia seed, cumin seed (if using), salt, and baking soda, and stir well. 3. Add the egg and olive oil to the dry ingredients and stir well until the dough forms a ball. 4. Cover the dough with parchment papers, using a rolling pin, roll the dough to ⅛-inch thickness, aiming for a rectangular shape. 5. Remove the parchment and, using a knife, cut the dough into 1- to 2-inch-square crackers. Transfer the cut cracker dough to a baking sheet. 6. Bake for 15 minutes, until crispy and slightly golden.

Per Serving: Calories 159; Total Fat 14g; Saturated Fat 1g; Sodium 262mg; Carbs 5g; Fiber 3g; Sugar 0g; Protein 6g

Keto Bread

Prep time: 2 minutes | Cook time: 2 minutes | Serves: 1 or 2

1 large egg
3 tablespoons almond flour
1 tablespoon extra-virgin olive oil

¼ teaspoon baking powder
¼ teaspoon salt

1. In a microwave-safe ramekin, mug, or small bowl, beat the egg. Add the almond flour, olive oil, baking powder, and salt, and mix well with a fork. 2. Microwave on high for 90 seconds. 3. Loosen the edges with help of knife of the ramekin and flip onto a plate or cutting board to remove the bread. Allow to cool for 2 minutes. 4. Slice the bread in half with a serrated knife.

Per Serving: Calories 318; Total Fat 29g; Saturated Fat 4g; Sodium 776mg; Carbs 5g; Fiber 2g; Sugar 9g; Protein 11g

Lime Beetroot Hummus

Prep Time: 10 minutes | Cook Time: 2 minutes |Serves: 2

1 (15-ounce) can chickpeas, drained and rinsed (save the water), plus more as needed
chickpea liquid)
1 cup cooked beetroot, canned or freshly cooked
1 garlic clove
2 tablespoons aquafaba (reserved canned chickpea

2 teaspoons extra-virgin olive oil
1 tablespoon tahini
1 tablespoon lime juice
½ teaspoon salt

1. The chickpeas, beetroot, garlic, aquafaba, oil, tahini, lime juice, and salt should be processed or blended to the appropriate consistency. 2. To thin down the hummus, add additional aquafaba if necessary.
Per Serving: Calories 139; Total Fat 6g; Saturated Fat 1g; Sodium 443mg; Carbs 19g; Fiber 5.2g; Sugar 6g; Protein 5g

Chocolate Cashew Raisins Truffles

Prep Time: 15 minutes | Cook Time: 0 minutes |Serves: 12

2 cups raisins
2 tablespoons water
1 cup raw cashews
1 tablespoon cocoa powder

1 teaspoon ground cinnamon
½ teaspoon vanilla extract
½ cup pumpkin seeds
¼ teaspoon salt

1. In a food processor, combine the raisins and water, and pulse until a paste forms. 2. In the food processor, combine the cashews, cocoa powder, cinnamon, and vanilla. Pulse just until a paste forms. 3. Once combined, add the salt and pumpkin seeds, and pulse until the seeds are finely minced. (Avoid over processing. The idea is to prevent the pumpkin seeds from becoming a paste.) 4. 2 teaspoons of the mixture should be scooped with a spoon and formed into little balls with your hands. Place on parchment paper with a 1-inch gap between each. 5. Keep in the refrigerator or at room temperature in an airtight container.

Per Serving: Calories 180; Total Fat 8g; Saturated Fat 1g; Sodium 553mg; Carbs 24g; Fiber 11g; Sugar 15.3g; Protein 10.4g

Cherry Chocolate Cashews Milkshake

Prep Time: 10 minutes | Cook Time: 0 minutes |Serves: 4

2 bananas, peeled or frozen (frozen make a creamier malt)
1½ cups frozen sweetened cherries
1 cup milk (dairy or plant-based)
1 cup ice cubes

½ cup raw cashews
½ cup coconut milk
2 tablespoons cocoa powder
2 teaspoons vanilla extract
2 teaspoons ground cinnamon (optional)

1. Bananas, cherries, dairy milk, ice cubes, cashews, coconut milk, cocoa powder, vanilla, and cinnamon (if used) should all be blended until smooth in a blender. 2. Pour into sealed jars for storage or serve right away. For three to four days in the freezer, the milkshake will stay fresh.

Per Serving: Calories 298; Total Fat 16g; Saturated Fat 8g; Sodium 123mg; Carbs 35g; Fiber 4.2g; Sugar 19g; Protein 8g

Soft Banana Cashew Ice Cream

Prep Time: 15 minutes | Cook Time: 0 minutes |Serves: 4

5 ripe bananas, frozen
¾ cup full-fat coconut milk
¼ cup cashew butter
2 teaspoons maple syrup (optional)

2 teaspoons vanilla extract
½ teaspoon ground cinnamon (optional)
½ cup dark chocolate chips or semisweet chocolate chips (optional)

1. Pulse the bananas, coconut milk, cashew butter, vanilla, maple syrup, and cinnamon in a food processor (if using). Process till creamy and smooth. The food processor should be pulsed five times after adding the chocolate chips (if using). 2. Serve right away or put in the freezer for up to 6 months in a freezer-safe container. Pour the ice-cream batter into the ice-pop moulds for simple storage and serving.

Per Serving: Calories 320; Total Fat 18g; Saturated Fat 10g; Sodium 223mg; Carbs 39g; Fiber 4.2g; Sugar 20g; Protein 4g

Nuts Date Bars

Prep Time: 10 minutes | Cook Time: 0 minutes |Serves: 12

1½ cups pitted Medjool dates
1 cup walnuts
½ cup almonds
¼ cup chia seeds

2 tablespoons unsweetened cocoa powder
1 teaspoon vanilla extract
⅛ teaspoon salt

1. Set aside an 8-inch square baking pan that has been lined with parchment paper. 2. The dates, walnuts, and almonds should all be combined in a powerful blender or food processor. The dates and nuts should be pulsed and processed until they disintegrate and begin to ball up. Add the salt, vanilla, cocoa powder, and chia seeds. Blend well after processing. 3. Press the mixture evenly onto the bottom of the baking pan after transferring it there. Place in the refrigerator for two hours, or until hard. For serving, divide into 12 bars. For up to a week, keep covered in the refrigerator.
Per Serving: Calories 170; Total Fat 10g; Saturated Fat 1g; Sodium 40mg; Carbs 19g; Fiber 12g; Sugar 5.3g; Protein 4.3g

Cheese Garlic Kale Chips

Prep Time: 5 minutes | Cook Time: 20 minutes |Serves: 4

1 bunch kale
1 tablespoon extra-virgin olive oil
3 garlic cloves, minced

¼ teaspoon salt
¼ cup finely shredded Parmesan cheese

1. Preheat the oven to 300°F. 2. After rinsing, pat the kale totally dry. The kale's ribs should be removed, and the leaves should be chopped finely and added to a big dish. Add salt, garlic, and olive oil before tossing. Spread the kale evenly and without crowding it onto a baking sheet. Make two batches if necessary. 3. While baking, toss the greens once after ten minutes. After the chips have had a chance to cool slightly, top them with Parmesan cheese. Serve right away. Any leftovers can be kept for up to five days in an airtight container.
Per Serving: Calories 80; Total Fat 5g; Saturated Fat 1g; Sodium 293mg; Carbs 4g; Fiber 1.2g; Sugar 1.3g; Protein 3.4g

Lime-Chili Popcorn

Prep Time: 5 minutes | Cook Time: 10 minutes |Serves: 8

1 tablespoon avocado oil
½ cup popcorn kernels
2 teaspoons chili powder

½ teaspoon salt
¼ teaspoon garlic powder
1 lime

1. Heat the avocado oil in a large, heavy saucepan over medium heat. Add the kernels of popcorn and cover with a lid. 2. For 6 to 7 minutes, reduce the heat and shake the pan intermittently to encourage all the kernels to pop and avoid scorching the ones that have already done so. Popcorn should continue to pop until the popping slows, at which point the pan should be taken off the heat while still being covered. 3. Throw away any unpopped kernels before transferring the popcorn to a big bowl. Add the grated lime zest to the popcorn along with the chile powder, salt, and garlic powder. 4. To ensure that the popcorn is uniformly covered, lightly toss it. Slice the lime in half just before serving, then squeeze the juice over the popcorn and toss to coat.
Per Serving: Calories 90; Total Fat 3g; Saturated Fat 0.5g; Sodium 263mg; Carbs 13.9g; Fiber 0.2g; Sugar 3.3g; Protein 2.14g

Rosemary Nuts Mix

Prep Time: 5 minutes | Cook Time: 20 minutes | Serves: 10

2½ cups unsalted mixed nuts
2 tablespoons pure maple syrup
1 tablespoon extra-virgin olive oil

2 tablespoons finely chopped fresh rosemary
¾ teaspoon salt
¼ teaspoon cayenne pepper

1. Preheat the oven to 350°F. Set aside a baking sheet that has been lined with parchment paper or a silicone baking mat. 2. The nuts, maple syrup, and olive oil should be combined in a big bowl. The nuts should be uniformly coated with the rosemary, salt, and cayenne pepper that have been added. Spread out the nuts evenly as you transfer them to the prepared baking sheet. 3. The nuts should be aromatic and brown after 15 to 20 minutes of baking, during which time they should be stirred twice. For up to a week, keep at room temperature in an airtight container.
Per Serving: Calories 226; Total Fat 19.3g; Saturated Fat 3.5g; Sodium 193mg; Carbs 11g; Fiber 3.2g; Sugar 3g; Protein 6g

Peanut Butter Flaxseed Balls

Prep Time: 10 minutes | Cook Time: 2 minutes | Serves: 20

1 cup natural peanut butter
½ cup peanut butter powder
½ cup ground flaxseed
2 tablespoons pure maple syrup

½ teaspoon vanilla extract
½ teaspoon ground cinnamon
⅛ teaspoon salt

1. Using a silicone spatula, thoroughly incorporate the peanut butter, peanut butter powder, flaxseed, vanilla, maple syrup, cinnamon, and salt in a medium bowl. 2. Roll a little amount of the mixture—about 1 tablespoon at a time—into a ball. Continue until all of the mixture has been shaped into balls. 3. For up to a week, keep in the refrigerator in an airtight container.
Per Serving: Calories 220; Total Fat 17.23g; Saturated Fat 3.5g; Sodium 123mg; Carbs 11.9g; Fiber 5.2g; Sugar 3.3g; Protein 11.4g

Peanut Butter Energy Balls

Prep time: 20 minutes | Cook time: 0 minutes | Serves: 12

1 cup unsweetened peanut or almond butter, stirred well
½ cup almond or coconut flour
¼ cup rolled quick-cooking oats
2 to 4 tablespoons granulated sugar-free sweetener

¼ cup unsweetened coconut flakes
¼ cup sugar-free chocolate chips, chopped
2 tablespoons chia seeds

1. In a bowl, add the peanut butter, almond flour, oats, sweetener to taste (if using), coconut flakes, chocolate chips, and chia seeds, mixing well with a fork or spoon. 2. Shape the mix into 12 balls, about 1 inch in diameter each. Transfer the energy balls to an airtight storage container, with a piece of parchment paper or waxed paper between each layer. The mixture will be sticky, but the balls will harden as they sit in the refrigerator. 3. Store covered in the refrigerator for up to 1week or the freezer for up to 3 months.
Per Serving: Calories 203; Total Fat 17g; Saturated Fat 4g; Sodium 5mg; Carbs 11g; Fiber 4g; Sugar 1g; Protein 7g

Nutty Cranberry Cereal Mix

Prep Time: 5 minutes | Cook Time: 15 minutes |Serves: 10

2 cups gluten-free whole-grain cereal
½ cup unsalted cashew halves
½ cup unsalted peanuts
½ cup unsweetened dried cranberries

½ cup golden raisins
⅔ cup natural creamy peanut butter
⅓ cup honey
½ teaspoon salt

1. Preheat the oven to 375°F. Set aside a baking sheet that has been lined with a parchment paper or a silicone baking mat. 2. Combine the cereal, cashews, peanuts, raisins and dried cranberries in a big bowl. Separate the mixture. 3. Combine the peanut butter, honey, and salt in a medium glass dish (or another vessel suitable for the microwave). Stirring every 20 to 30 seconds, microwave on high for 1 minute, or until the peanut butter is melted. Pour the peanut butter mixture over the cereal-nut mixture after thoroughly combining it. Until everything is well covered, stir. Spread the mixture evenly across the entire baking sheet as you pour it onto the prepared sheet. 4. When the coating is set, bake for another 15 minutes, stirring every five minutes. Allow the mixture to cool. Store it in an airtight container for up to 1 week.
Per Serving: Calories 290; Total Fat 16g; Saturated Fat 5g; Sodium 163mg; Carbs 35g; Fiber 21g; Sugar 3.3g; Protein 8g

Coconut Oats Cookies

Prep time: 5 minutes | Cook time: 15 minutes | Serves: 16

¾ cup almond flour
¾ cup old-fashioned oats
¼ cup shredded unsweetened coconut
1 teaspoon baking powder
1 teaspoon ground cinnamon

¼ teaspoon salt
¼ cup unsweetened applesauce
1 large egg
1 tablespoon pure maple syrup
2 tablespoons coconut oil, melted

1. Preheat the oven to 350°F temp setting. 2. In a medium mixing bowl, combine the almond flour, oats, coconut, baking powder, cinnamon, and salt, and mix well. 3. In another medium bowl, combine the maple syrup, applesauce, egg, and coconut oil, and mix. Stir the wet mixture into the dry mixture. 4. Form the dough into balls a little bigger than a tablespoon and place on a baking sheet, leaving at least 1 inch between them. Bake for 12 minutes until browned. Let cool for 5 minutes. 5. Using a spatula, remove the cookies and cool on a rack.
Per Serving: Calories 76; Total Fat 6g; Saturated Fat 0.2g; Sodium 57mg; Carbs 5g; Fiber 1g; Sugar 2g; Protein 2g

Butter Pecan Cookies

Prep time: 10 minutes | Cook time: 20 minutes | Serves: 12

½ cup (1 stick) unsalted butter
½ cup granulated sugar-free sweetener, such as Swerve
1 large egg
1 teaspoon vanilla extract
2 cups almond flour

1 teaspoon xanthan gum
½ teaspoon baking powder
½ teaspoon ground cinnamon
1 cup chopped pecans

1. Preheat the oven to 350°F. Manage a baking sheet with parchment paper. 2. In a bowl, using an electric mixer on medium speed, cream together the butter and sweetener until smooth. Add the egg along with vanilla and beat well, scraping down the sides of the bowl as needed. 3. Add the almond flour, xanthan gum, baking powder, and cinnamon, and stir with a wooden spoon or spatula until well incorporated. Stir in the pecans. 4. Using a tablespoon, spoon 2-tablespoon mounds of dough, about 1 inch apart, on the prepared baking sheet. 5. Bake the cookies for 18 minutes, until set and lightly golden. Let sit on the baking sheet for 10 minutes. Then transfer to a cooling rack and serve.

Per Serving: Calories 246; Total Fat 24g; Saturated Fat 6g; Sodium 31mg; Carbs 13g; Fiber 3g; Sugar 8g; Protein 5g

Chapter 8 Sauces, Dips, and Dressings Recipes

Lemon Parsley Yogurt Sauce

Prep time: 10 minutes | Cook time: 0 minutes | Serves: 1 ½ cups

½ cup Italian parsley leaves
1 garlic clove
1 cup full-fat plain Greek yogurt
¼ cup extra-virgin olive oil

¼ cup freshly squeezed lemon juice
1 teaspoon salt
¼ teaspoon freshly ground black pepper

1. Combine the parsley with garlic in a food processor and pulse until well chopped. 2. Add the yogurt with olive oil, lemon juice, salt, and black pepper, and pulse until smooth and creamy. 3. Store in an airtight container in the refrigerator for up to 1 week.

Per Serving: Calories 117; Total Fat 11g; Saturated Fat 2g; Sodium 411mg; Carbs 2g; Fiber 0.1g; Sugar 0g; Protein 4g

Easy Coconut Cream Sauce

Prep time: 5 minutes | Cook time: 10 minutes | Serves: ½ cup

1 tablespoon unsalted butter
1 tablespoon flour
¼ teaspoon sea salt

Pinch of white pepper
1 cup coconut cream

1. In a medium-sized heavy nonstick saucepan, melt the butter over very low heat. Butter should gently melt; you do not want it to bubble and turn brown. 2. While the butter melts, mix the flour, salt, and white pepper in a small bowl. 3. Add the flour mixture in butter, stirring constantly. 4. Once mixture thickens and starts to bubble, about 2 minutes, slowly pour in one-third of the coconut cream; stir until blended with roux. Add another one-third coconut cream; stir until blended. Add remaining coconut cream and continue cooking, stirring constantly to make sure sauce doesn't stick to bottom of pan. Once sauce begins to steam and appears it's just about to boil, reduce heat and simmer until sauce thickens, or about 3 minutes.

Per Serving: Calories 61; Total Fat 3g; Saturated Fat 2g; Sodium 190mg; Carbs 6g; Fiber 0g; Sugar 0g; Protein 2g

Lemon-Garlic Hummus

Prep time: 15 minutes | Cook time: 0 minutes | Serves: 8

1 (15 ounce) can no-salt-added chickpeas, drained (liquid reserved) and rinsed
¼ cup ground flaxseed
2 tablespoons olive oil
2 tablespoons freshly squeezed lemon juice

3 garlic cloves, peeled
½ teaspoon ground cumin
½ teaspoon salt
½ teaspoon sesame oil

1. Place the chickpeas and ¼ cup of the reserved liquid, flaxseed, olive oil, lemon juice, garlic, cumin powder, salt, and sesame oil in a processor. Process until smooth and creamy. Pour in additional reserved bean liquid until it reaches your desired consistency. 2. Transfer the hummus to a bowl. Drizzle with additional olive oil and serve. 3. Store in an airtight container in the refrigerator for up to 7 days.

Per Serving: Calories 108; Total Fat 6g; Saturated Fat 1g; Sodium 149mg; Carbs 10g; Fiber 3g; Sugar 2g; Protein 4g

Cheesy Basil Pine Nuts Sauce

Prep time: 5 minutes | Cook time: 0 minutes | Serves: 1 cup

2 cups fresh basil leaves
½ cup extra-virgin olive oil
½ cup finely shredded Parmesan cheese
¼ cup pine nuts

3 garlic cloves, peeled
2 tablespoons freshly squeezed lemon juice
¼ teaspoon salt
¼ freshly ground black pepper

1. Put the basil, olive oil, Parmesan, pine nuts, garlic, lemon juice, salt, and pepper in a food processor on high for 45 to 60 seconds or until it reaches a smooth consistency. Serve. 2. Store in an airtight container in the refrigerator for up to 5 day or in the freezer for 3 to 4 months.
Per Serving: Calories 178; Total Fat 18g; Saturated Fat 3g; Sodium 186mg; Carbs 2g; Fiber 0g; Sugar 0g; Protein 3g

Sweet-and-Sour Sauce

Prep time: 5 minutes | Cook time: 10 minutes | Serves: 1 ¼ cups

½ cup 100% pineapple juice
⅓ cup apple cider vinegar
⅓ cup ketchup
3 Medjool dates, pitted

2 garlic cloves, peeled
2 tablespoons water
1 tablespoon reduced-sodium tamari
2 teaspoons cornstarch

1. Put the pineapple juice, apple cider vinegar, ketchup, dates, garlic, water, tamari, and cornstarch in a blender. Blend it for 2 minutes, or until it forms a smooth, uniform consistency. 2. Transfer the sauce to a saucepan over medium-high heat. Boil on low heat, stirring constantly, until the sauce has darkened and slightly thickened, about 10 minutes. Serve.
Per Serving: Calories 40; Total Fat 0g; Saturated Fat 0g; Sodium 124mg; Carbs 10g; Fiber 1g; Sugar 8g; Protein 0g

Raspberry Vinaigrette

Prep time: 5 minutes | Cook time: 0 minutes | Serves: 1 cup

¾ cup avocado oil
¼ cup red wine vinegar
¼ cup fresh raspberries
1 tablespoon honey

¼ teaspoon paprika
⅛ teaspoon salt
⅛ teaspoon freshly ground black pepper

1. Put the oil, vinegar, raspberries, honey, paprika, salt, and pepper in a blender. Puree until it reaches a smooth consistency, 30 to 60 seconds. Serve. 2. Refrigerate in a sealed container for up to 7 days.
Per Serving: Calories 192; Total Fat 20g; Saturated Fat 3g; Sodium 40mg; Carbs 3g; Fiber 0g; Sugar 2g; Protein 0g

Homemade Apple Cider Vinaigrette Dressing

Prep time: 5 minutes | Cook time: 0 minutes | Serves: 2/3 cup

⅓ cup extra-virgin olive oil
¼ cup apple cider vinegar
2 teaspoons honey
2 teaspoons Dijon mustard

1 garlic clove, minced
⅛ teaspoon freshly ground black pepper
⅛ teaspoon salt

1. Put the oil, vinegar, honey, mustard, garlic, salt and pepper in a small jar, cover, and shake until well blended. Serve. 2. Refrigerate for up to 1 week. Shake the dressing well to recombine ingredients before using.
Per Serving: Calories 139; Total Fat 14g; Saturated Fat 2g; Sodium 85mg; Carbs 3g; Fiber 0g; Sugar 2g; Protein 0g

Creamy Chipotle-Lime Dressing

Prep time: 5 minutes | Cook time: 0 minutes | Serves: 1 cup

¾ cup plain nonfat Greek yogurt
1 chipotle pepper
1 to 2 teaspoons adobo sauce
1 tablespoon freshly squeezed lime juice
1 teaspoon grated lime zest

1 garlic clove, peeled
½ teaspoon smoked paprika
¼ teaspoon salt
¼ teaspoon freshly ground black pepper

1. Put the yogurt, chipotle pepper, adobo sauce, lime juice, lime zest, garlic, paprika, salt, and pepper in a blender or food processor. Blend for 30 seconds until creamy. Serve. 2. Use as a salad dressing, a topping for tacos, nachos, or power bowls, a condiment in your sandwich or wrap, or as a dip for chicken strips or baked sweet potatoes.
Per Serving: Calories 16; Total Fat 0g; Saturated Fat 0g; Sodium 81mg; Carbs 2g; Fiber 0g; Sugar 1g; Protein 2g

Yogurt Dill Sauce

Prep time: 5 minutes | Cook time: 0 minutes | Serves: 1 cup

1 cup plain nonfat Greek yogurt
1½ tablespoons freshly squeezed lemon juice
1 tablespoon dried dill weed or 2 tablespoons

chopped fresh dill
¼ teaspoon salt
¼ teaspoon freshly ground black pepper

1. In a bowl, whisk the yogurt with the lemon juice, dill, salt, and pepper until well blended. Serve. 2. Refrigerate in a sealed jar or container for up to 1 week.
Per Serving: Calories 18; Total Fat 0g; Saturated Fat 0g; Sodium 84mg; Carbs 1g; Fiber 0g; Sugar 1g; Protein 3g

Lemon Vinaigrette Dressing

Prep time: 5-10 minutes | Cook time: 0 minutes | Serves: 1 cup

¼ cup freshly squeezed lemon juice
2 garlic cloves, minced
1 teaspoon Dijon mustard
½ teaspoon maple syrup (optional)

¼ cup extra-virgin olive oil
½ cup grapeseed oil
Kosher salt
Freshly ground black pepper

1. In a bowl, combine the lemon juice, garlic, mustard, and maple syrup (if using). Slowly whisk in the extra-virgin olive oil, followed by the grapeseed oil, until the dressing is completely emulsified. Spice with salt and pepper. 2. Store the dressing in an airtight container for up to 1 week in the refrigerator or in the freezer for up to 3 months.

Per Serving: Calories 184; Total Fat 20g; Saturated Fat 0.8g; Sodium 122mg; Carbs 1g; Fiber 0.2g; Sugar 0.2g; Protein 0.9g

Spicy Lime Salad Dressing

Prep time: 5 minutes | Cook time: 0 minutes | Serves: 1 cup

5 ounces grapeseed or safflower oil
Zest and juice of 4 limes
4 garlic cloves, minced
4-inch piece fresh ginger, minced

2½ tablespoons chile paste
2 teaspoons fish sauce (optional)
¼ teaspoon kosher salt

1. Combine the grapeseed oil, lime zest and juice, garlic, ginger, chile paste, fish sauce (if using), and salt in a jar or container with a tight-fitting lid. Close the lid and shake the mixture vigorously to combine. 2. Store the dressing in an airtight container for up to 1 week in the refrigerator or in the freezer for up to 3 months.

Per Serving: Calories 179; Total Fat 18g; Saturated Fat 0.6g; Sodium 159mg; Carbs 6g; Fiber 0.2g; Sugar 0.2g; Protein 0.9g

Cilantro Guacamole

Prep Time: 10 minutes | Cook Time: 0 minutes | Serves: 6

2 large avocados
1 small, firm tomato, finely diced
¼ white onion, finely diced
¼ cup finely chopped fresh cilantro

2 tablespoons freshly squeezed lime juice
¼ teaspoon salt
Freshly ground black pepper

1. Halve the avocados, scoop out the flesh into a medium dish, and discard the seeds. 2. Mash the avocado flesh with a fork. Add the salt, lime juice, cilantro, tomato, and onion to the mixture. Use black pepper to season. 3. Serve right away.

Per Serving: Calories 90; Total Fat 7g; Saturated Fat 1.5g; Sodium 183mg; Carbs 6g; Fiber 1.2g; Sugar 3.3g; Protein 1.4g

Red Beet-Yogurt Dip

Prep Time: 10 minutes | Cook Time: 60 minutes |Serves: 6

½ pound red beets
½ cup plain nonfat Greek yogurt
1 tablespoon extra-virgin olive oil
1 tablespoon freshly squeezed lemon juice

1 garlic clove, peeled
1 teaspoon minced fresh thyme
½ teaspoon onion powder
¼ teaspoon salt

1. Turn the oven on to 375°F. Bake the beets for 45 to 60 minutes, or until they are tender when pricked with a fork, wrapped in aluminium foil. 2. Place aside and allow it cool for a minimum of 10 minutes. Remove the beets' skins with your hands, then add them to a blender. 3. Yogurt, olive oil, lemon juice, garlic, thyme, onion powder, and salt should all be added to the blender jar. until smooth, process. One hour should pass before serving.

Per Serving: Calories 50; Total Fat 2.3g; Saturated Fat 0.5g; Sodium 143mg; Carbs 5g; Fiber 3.2g; Sugar 1.33g; Protein 3.4g

Cucumber-Yogurt Dip

Prep Time: 10 minutes | Cook Time: 0 minutes |Serves: 6

1 medium cucumber, peeled and grated
¼ teaspoon salt
1 cup plain nonfat Greek yogurt
2 garlic cloves, minced

1 tablespoon freshly squeezed lemon juice
1 tablespoon extra-virgin olive oil
¼ teaspoon freshly ground black pepper

1. Place the cucumber in a sieve and season with salt. Place aside. 2. Mix the yogurt, garlic, lemon juice, olive oil, and pepper in a medium bowl. 3. Squeeze as much water as you can from the shredded cucumber using your hands. Stir well after adding the cucumber to the yogurt mixture. If desired, cover and chill for two hours to allow the flavors to meld. 4. For up to five to seven days, keep in the refrigerator in an airtight container.

Per Serving: Calories 50; Total Fat 3g; Saturated Fat 0.5g; Sodium 113mg; Carbs 3.9g; Fiber 2g; Sugar 0.33g; Protein 4g

Flavorful Caramelized Onion-Yogurt Dip

Prep Time: 10 minutes | Cook Time: 45 minutes |Serves: 8

2 tablespoons extra-virgin olive oil
3 cups chopped onions
1 garlic clove, minced

2 cups plain nonfat Greek yogurt
1 teaspoon salt
Freshly ground black pepper

1. Olive oil should be heated to shimmering condition in a big saucepan over medium heat. Stir carefully to coat the onions after adding them. When well-browned and caramelized, reduce heat to low, cover, and simmer for 45 minutes, stirring every 5 to 10 minutes. Stir in the garlic until it is barely aromatic. 2. After 10 minutes, turn off the heat and let the food cool. 3. Combine the onions, yogurt, salt, and pepper in a mixing dish.

Per Serving: Calories 85; Total Fat 4g; Saturated Fat 1g; Sodium 223mg; Carbs 7g; Fiber 5g; Sugar 1.3g; Protein 6.4g

Ginger-Garlic Miso Dressing

Prep Time: 10 minutes | Cook Time: 0 minutes |Serves: 4

1 tablespoon unseasoned rice vinegar
1 tablespoon red or white miso
1 teaspoon grated fresh ginger

1 garlic clove, minced
3 tablespoons extra-virgin olive oil

1. Make a paste out of the miso and vinegar in a small basin. Mix thoroughly after adding the ginger and garlic. Add the olive oil in a thin stream while whisking. 2. For up to a week, keep in the refrigerator in an airtight container.

Per Serving: Calories 100; Total Fat 10g; Saturated Fat 1g; Sodium 223mg; Carbs 1g; Fiber 0g; Sugar 0g; Protein 1.4g

Italian Red Wine Vinegar Dressing

Prep Time: 5 minutes | Cook Time: 0 minutes |Serves: 12

¼ cup red wine vinegar
½ cup extra-virgin olive oil
¼ teaspoon salt
¼ teaspoon freshly ground black pepper

1 teaspoon dried Italian seasoning
1 teaspoon Dijon mustard
1 garlic clove, minced

1. Combine the mustard, garlic, salt, pepper, Italian seasoning, vinegar, and olive oil in a small container. Put a tight-fitting cover on top and shake ferociously for one minute. 2. Keep chilled for up to a week.

Per Serving: Calories 80; Total Fat 9g; Saturated Fat 0g; Sodium 83mg; Carbs 0g; Fiber 0g; Sugar 0g; Protein 0g

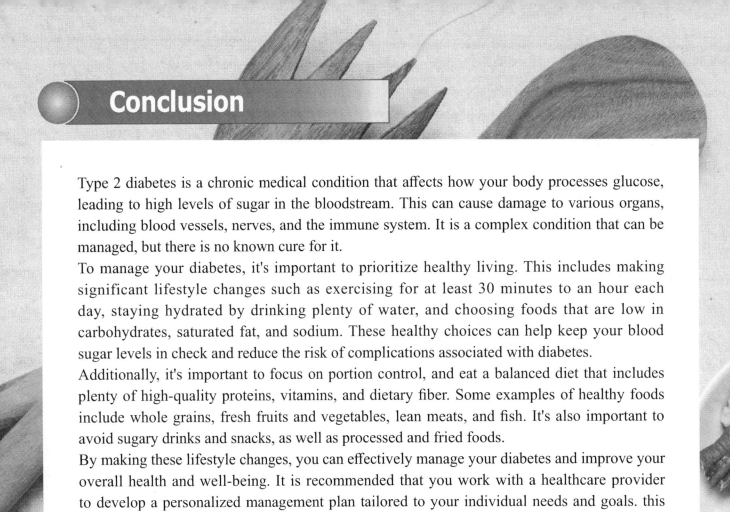

Conclusion

Type 2 diabetes is a chronic medical condition that affects how your body processes glucose, leading to high levels of sugar in the bloodstream. This can cause damage to various organs, including blood vessels, nerves, and the immune system. It is a complex condition that can be managed, but there is no known cure for it.

To manage your diabetes, it's important to prioritize healthy living. This includes making significant lifestyle changes such as exercising for at least 30 minutes to an hour each day, staying hydrated by drinking plenty of water, and choosing foods that are low in carbohydrates, saturated fat, and sodium. These healthy choices can help keep your blood sugar levels in check and reduce the risk of complications associated with diabetes.

Additionally, it's important to focus on portion control, and eat a balanced diet that includes plenty of high-quality proteins, vitamins, and dietary fiber. Some examples of healthy foods include whole grains, fresh fruits and vegetables, lean meats, and fish. It's also important to avoid sugary drinks and snacks, as well as processed and fried foods.

By making these lifestyle changes, you can effectively manage your diabetes and improve your overall health and well-being. It is recommended that you work with a healthcare provider to develop a personalized management plan tailored to your individual needs and goals. this cookbook is the best to journal for your diet management to maintain a healthy lifestyle. With proper care and control, it is possible to live a healthy and fulfilling life with type 2 diabetes.

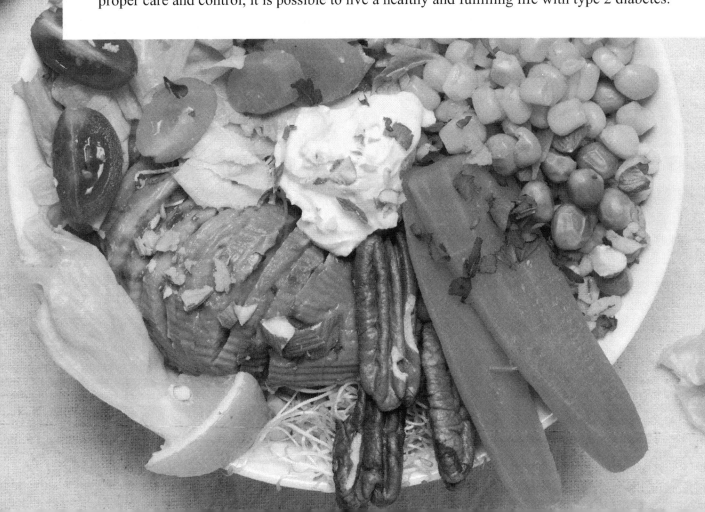

Appendix 1 Measurement Conversion Chart

VOLUME EQUIVALENTS (LIQUID)

US STANDARD	US STANDARD (OUNCES)	METRIC (APPROXIMATE)
2 tablespoons	1 fl.oz	30 mL
¼ cup	2 fl.oz	60 mL
½ cup	4 fl.oz	120 mL
1 cup	8 fl.oz	240 mL
1½ cup	12 fl.oz	355 mL
2 cups or 1 pint	16 fl.oz	475 mL
4 cups or 1 quart	32 fl.oz	1 L
1 gallon	128 fl.oz	4 L

TEMPERATURES EQUIVALENTS

FAHRENHEIT (F)	CELSIUS(C) (APPROXIMATE)
225 °F	107 °C
250 °F	120 °C
275 °F	135 °C
300 °F	150 °C
325 °F	160 °C
350 °F	180 °C
375 °F	190 °C
400 °F	205 °C
425 °F	220 °C
450 °F	235 °C
475 °F	245 °C
500 °F	260 °C

VOLUME EQUIVALENTS (DRY)

US STANDARD	METRIC (APPROXIMATE)
⅛ teaspoon	0.5 mL
¼ teaspoon	1 mL
½ teaspoon	2 mL
¾ teaspoon	4 mL
1 teaspoon	5 mL
1 tablespoon	15 mL
¼ cup	59 mL
½ cup	118 mL
¾ cup	177 mL
1 cup	235 mL
2 cups	475 mL
3 cups	700 mL
4 cups	1 L

VOLUME EQUIVALENTS (DRY)

US STANDARD	METRIC (APPROXIMATE)
1 ounce	28 g
2 ounces	57 g
5 ounces	142 g
10 ounces	284 g
15 ounces	425 g
16 ounces (1 pound)	455 g
1.5 pounds	680 g
2 pounds	907 g

Appendix 2 Recipes Index

Made in the USA
Monee, IL
04 April 2025

15165701R00065